T0144753

Assessment of Quality of Life for Cancer Patients

Cancer is a deadly disease that puts not only physical and financial pressure on the patient but also even more psychological pressure. Physical deterioration in health and financial losses are easy to see, but the psychological effects are not as visible; however, the psychological aspects are an important component in measuring any patient's quality of life (QoL, or balance between physical, psychological, social, and spiritual components).

The present study is a small step in the direction of measuring QoL of cancer patients and the potential positive impact of changes in counselling. The association between QoL and other parameters, especially fear, leads to the recommendation to set up counselling centres at each hospital in its oncology department.

Alpana Srivastava, PhD (Statistics), MBA (Operation Management), MSc (Statistics), MA (Economics), BSc, is Professor and Area Head (Statistics, Economics, IT & Operation Management) at Amity Business School, Amity University, Lucknow, Uttar Pradesh, India, and President of ASEDS, India.

Assessment of Quality of Life for Cancer Patients

Lessons from a Study in a Tertiary Care Hospital in Uttar Pradesh, India

Prof. (Dr.) Alpana Srivastava
Amity Business School
Amity University, Uttar Pradesh
Lucknow, India

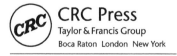

CRC Press
Taylor & Francis Group
Boca Raton London New York

CRC Press is an imprint of the
Taylor & Francis Group, an **informa** business

Designed cover image: Author

First edition published 2024
by CRC Press
2385 NW Executive Center Drive, Suite 320, Boca Raton FL 33431

and by CRC Press
4 Park Square, Milton Park, Abingdon, Oxon, OX14 4RN

CRC Press is an imprint of Taylor & Francis Group, LLC

© 2024 Alpana Srivastava

ISBN: 9781032571393 (hbk)
ISBN: 9781032571386 (pbk)
ISBN: 9781003437994 (ebk)

DOI: 10.1201/9781003437994

Typeset in Caslon
by Apex CoVantage, LLC

To my beloved mother,

In the face of the greatest adversity, your unwavering
courage and indomitable spirit have shone brighter
than any star. This book is dedicated to you, my source
of strength, and an inspiration beyond measure.

As you battle this relentless foe with grace and resilience, I
am reminded of the countless others who face this formidable
adversary called cancer. Through this book, may we shed
light on the darkness of this disease, and may it serve
as a beacon of hope for those in their own battles.

Your fight is my motivation, and your love is my driving force.
I dedicate this book to you, Mom, and to all the brave souls
who confront cancer with unwavering determination.

your loving daughter, Alpana.

Contents

Tables

Figures

Acknowledgements

The project on which this text is based was conducted in a time period extended to 12 months and took endeavours and efforts from many people and institutions.

First of all, I would like to express my heartfelt thanks to the Indian Council of Social Science Research (ICSSR) for considering the importance of this social cum health care necessity for the society at a broader level and sponsoring the project for the social cause.

I'm extremely thankful to Dr Sunil Dhanshwar (Pro VC, AUUP) for providing institutional support and infrastructural requirements. Also, I would like to express my gratitude to Dr Rohit Kushawa (Director, Amity Business School) for consistent support throughout the project.

Dr Sandeep Tiwari, HoD Trauma Surgery Department, KGMU, Dr Gyan Chandra (SGPGI) and Dr Shaswat (RML) deserve special thanks as nodal officers for the project and helped a lot in recording patient information and providing their valuable input and insights periodically. Dr Tiwari also helped in obtaining ethical clearance for this study.

My thanks are also due to Dr Rajiv Gupta (Prof. and Head Radiology, KGMU), Dr Amit Pandey (KGMU), Dr Vajai Arora (KGMU) and Dr Rahat Hadi (Radiation Oncology, RML) for their help in ensuring interviews with their patients.

My thanks are due to Dr Deepak Ohri (Dean Research, AUUP) and Dr Sunila Dhaneshwar (Dy. Dean Research, AUUP) for their constant and consistent administrative support throughout the project's tenure. Dr Nimish Gupta (Assoc. Prof. AUUP) has always extended his support through all possible means, and throughout the project he was available for all kinds of technical support.

I express my gratitude to Mr Suhel Ahmad and Miss Tanu Tiwari, research scholars at AUUP, who worked as field executives for the project and collected the data from different hospitals and prepared the data for the analysis. Mr Sanjiv Srivastava, a research scholar at AUUP, also helped a lot in bridging all kinds of associations with KGMU, Lucknow.

Last, but not least, I express my thanks to the Accounts Department (AUUP) for prompt release of funds as and when required and Amity Central Library for ensuring and availing various required books and texts. The Procurement Department (AUUP) and IT Department (AUUP) also deserve to be mentioned here for their help and support in various purchases and technical help, respectively.

I once again thank all those people and institutions involved in this project. Without your support, this work could not have been realised.

Thank you!

Prof. (Dr.) Alpana Srivastava

Introduction

Cancer is a deadly disease, and it not only puts physical and financial pressure but also psychological pressure on the sufferer. It is seen that physical deterioration in health and financial losses are easily visible, but the psychological corrosions are not as easily seen. A number of research studies in developed nations suggest a positive correlation between quality of life (QoL) and this neglected parameter, but in India we have made negligible effort in this direction. QoL is considered to be the vital health outcome measure for a cancer patient's care. It is a term incorporating various aspects of life such as physical, psychological, socio-economical, spiritual, cognitional and social dimensions. Balance between all the four domains (i.e. physical, psychological, social and spiritual) means a good QoL. The present study is a small step in this area. Uttar Pradesh (UP) was the area used for the study. UP is the highest-populated state in India with an inadequate health infrastructure. Most of the tertiary care hospitals in UP are centred at Lucknow. The data is collected from three tertiary care hospitals located in Lucknow district, viz: King George Medical University (KGMU), Sanjay Gandhi Post Graduate Institute of Medical Sciences (SGPGIMS), and Dr Ram Manohar Lohia (Dr RML) Hospital. The sample size was around 300. A tested instrument of Ferrell's QOL is used for measuring QoL of the cancer patients. The findings support that mostly a low-income group are visiting these hospitals as opposed to those with a higher income, hence the QoL of the majority of patients is below average at the initial stage only. QoL scores are in general very low: 29.16% of the respondents have less than 0.5 on QoL indexes, which is of great concern. Only 2.89% have an index more than 0.6. Thus we see that much help is needed at the micro level and the macro level to overcome this great problem and ensure for each patient a good QoL. Post follow-up saw a slight change in the QoL scores: 37.21% of the respondents had less than a 0.6 score, which was a big change in the follow-up survey cases, as 13.91% were below 0.7 and 1.13 were greater than 0.7. Thus we see that a small effort was able to bring a slight change in ensuring for each patient a good QoL; hence, we should propose proper counselling of these patients to bring a change in the QoL index.

Fear has been factored out as one important parameter in the psychological domain responsible for low QoL. The highest fear factor was of recurrence (89.1%) and spreading (89.4%). A reported 87.5% feared a second cancer, while 84.9% were afraid of future test results as well. This study, first of its kind for UP, clearly brings out the association between QoL and other parameters, especially fear; hence, the author recommends setting up counselling centres at each hospital in the oncology department for increasing the QoL of cancer patients.

CHAPTER 1

Portrayal of the Study

1.1 Introduction

Among several diseases, cancer has become a big threat to human beings globally. Cancer is a presently prominent cause of morbidity and mortality universally, with approximately 14.1 million new cases and 8.2 million cancer-related deaths in 2012 and a 5-year prevalence of 32.6 million cancers in individuals above the age of 15 years as reported by the International Agency for Research on Cancer (IARC, 2014). The report also indicates a substantive increase in 19.3 million new cancer patients by 2025. The most commonly occurring cancers in men are cancers of the lung, prostate, colorectal, stomach, and liver which amounts to a total of 4.3 million cancer cases, whereas in women, the most common cancers are breast followed by colorectal, lung, and cervix and corpus uteri that amounts to a total of 3.7 million cases reported globally.

Demographic and epidemiological transitions are the two main population changes happening in countries around the world, and they generally go hand in hand. With economic development, countries reduce their birth and death rates, and the population pyramid becomes rectangular i.e. the aging population increases while the number of children and young decreases on one hand and also, with economic development, infectious diseases are slowly replaced by chronic diseases. The effects of these two transitions are reflected on the cancer rates as well. In India as we have a smaller aging population and a larger young population, the incidence rates of cancer are low as compared to other nations. But seeing its huge population, cancer is considered to be the second most common disease which is responsible for maximum mortality, with about 0.3 million deaths per year in India. This is owing to the poor availability of prevention, diagnosis, poverty, and low affordability of treatment for the disease. The main causes of such high incidence rates of most type of cancers may be both internal (genetic, mutations, hormonal, poor immune conditions) and external or environmental factors (food habits, industrialisation, overgrowth of the population, social, etc.).

Cancer is a major cause of morbidity and mortality in developing and developed nations both. The main reason behind this is that in many low-income and middle-income countries, including India, the majority of the population suffering from this deadly disease do not have access to a well-organised and well-regulated cancer care system. A diagnosis of cancer often leads to catastrophic personal health expenditures along with pushing the entire family below the poverty line by an over-increase in expenditures. This, when combined with an absence of efficient and acceptable services, threatens individual well-being, family well-being, and social well-being, bringing social instability. Population ageing is often assumed to be the main factor driving increases in cancer incidence, death rates, and health care costs, but the actual picture is more complex. In high-income countries age-standardised cancer mortality is now typically decreasing in all age groups, although more than half of all cancer-related deaths are among people older than 70 years. In India, despite the weakness of data in terms of population coverage, no evidence exists for a decrease in age-standardised cancer mortality rates, and most deaths occur in individuals younger than 70 years. These differences may be because of our young demographic population as compared to other countries. Poor access to screening and early-stage case-finding services also helps to explain the paradox of India's seemingly low cancer incidence rates but relatively high age-specific death rates.

The situation in India is also alarming as cancer is spreading like an epidemic. India is likely to have over 17.3 lakh new cases of cancer and over 8.8 lakh deaths due to the disease by 2020, with cancers of the breast, lung, and cervix topping the list. A premier medical research body, the Indian Council of Medical Research (ICMR), cited this information in its report. In its projection, they said that in 2016 the total number of new cancer cases is expected to be around 14.5 lakh, and the figure is likely to reach nearly 17.3 lakh new cases in 2020. Over 7.36 lakh people are expected to succumb to the disease in 2016, while the figure is estimated to shoot up to 8.8 lakh by 2020. Data also revealed that only 12.5% of patients come for treatment in early stages of the disease and the rest generally come at the advance stage. The risk of getting cancer before age 75 is 10.1% in India, which is also alarming. Life expectancy, demographic transitions, effects of tobacco, and other risk factors of modern life-styles will further increase the burden of cancer in the coming years.

Uttar Pradesh (UP) is the highest populated state in India with an inadequate health infrastructure. Most of the tertiary care hospitals in UP are centred at Lucknow. Tertiary care is specialized consultative health care, usually provided for in-patients following from primary or secondary health professionals, in an institution that has personnel and facilities for advanced laboratory and imaging investigations as well as for highly skilled clinical management. In the case of cancer, patients generally report their disease at an advanced stage and hence are referred to tertiary care hospitals. Considering the population pressures, these centres cannot cater to all the referred patients, and those catered to are mainly provided with basic treatment. Psychological, socio-economical, spiritual, cognitional, and social dimensions, due to various constraints, are not given due importance. But it is seen by various researches globally that if all these factors are considered as a part of cancer treatment, a longer life span could be ensured. Hence, today more emphasis is given to measure the quality of life (QoL) of the patients in general and cancer patients in particular.

No national registry exists that provides comprehensive cancer incidence or mortality data for India. However, the National Cancer Registry Programme (NCRP, established by the ICMR in 1981) provides population-based data from a selected network of 28 cancer registries located across the country.

An alarming fact was reported by the Boston Consulting Group Study, that nearly 60–80% of cancer cases in India are diagnosed late, and 60% patients do not have access to quality treatment as given in Figure 1. There are only 300-plus cancer centres in India, while the demand is for 600 and more. Only 400 radiotherapy machines are available, whereas the requirement is for more than 1200 to cover the cancer population adequately. Moreover, it is also reported that about 40% of centres are not equipped

	Incident cases	Deaths	Incidence ASR	Mortality ASR	Mortality to Incidence ratio
Very high HDI	5780821	2606104	279.2	105.3	37.7
High HDI	2126439	1244496	180.2	102.3	56.8
Medium HDI	5232474	3656562	144.2	102.8	70.9
Low HDI	943102	690141	112.8	86.7	76.9
India	1014934	682830	94.0	64.5	68.6

FIGURE 1 Cancer incidence and mortality in India in very high, high, medium, and low development index regions, 2012. HDI, human development index; ASR, age-standardised rate, adjusted for world population and in 100,000 population.

Source: Mallath et al., 2014, with permission.

with all modern facilities. They also estimated that India needs 500 positron emission tomography–computed tomography (PET-CT) machines and 1000 cancer units by year 2020 with the present pace of increase in cancer patients. The doctor-patient ratio is 1:2000, and the current aim is to achieve 1:1000 by 2021.There is also disproportionate skilful manpower and technology in India with cancer specialists, trained staff, and specialised cancer centres available in very few cities across India. Figure 2,

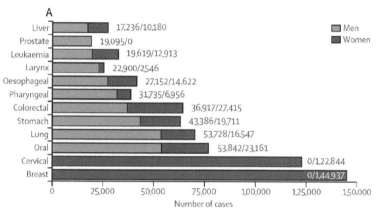

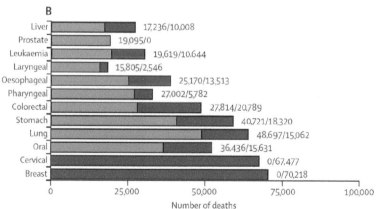

FIGURE 2 Incidence (A), mortality (B), and prevalence (C) of the most common cancers in Indian men and women in 2012.

Source: Mallath et al., 2014, with permission.

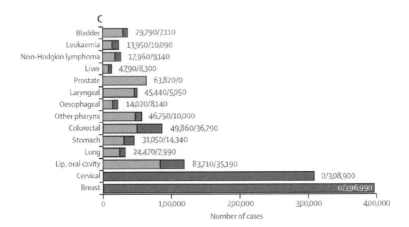

FIGURE 2 (Continued)

(A B & C) shows the scenario of incidence, mortality and prevalance of cancer in men and women in India a decade ago as reported by Mallath et al., 2014.

As most of the population is from a lower-income group, they do not have insurance coverage, and the cost of treatment is out of their reach. Thus we see that in India quality and affordable cancer care is a big challenge. Its diagnosis causes immense emotional trauma, and its treatment is a major economic burden. At the initial stage of diagnosis of cancer, it is perceived by many patients as a grave event with more than one-third of them suffering from high anxiety and depression, thus leading to a worse QoL. Cancer is equally distressing for the family and job environment. It also affects both a family's daily functioning and economic situation. The economic shock includes both loss of income and increase of expenses because of treatment and health care. This disease is associated with a lot of fear, misery, and isolation in our country.

The success or failure of any hospital largely depends on the satisfaction of the patients in terms of various services

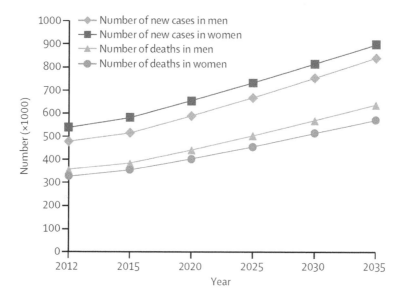

FIGURE 3 Estimated projected incidence and mortality burden of all cancers in Indian men and women to 2035.

Source: Mallath et al., 2014, with permission.

offered. With the various changes and developments that take place in a health care–related environment, patients place more importance on the quality of services offered than ever before. In recent days patients emphasise not only the environment in the hospitals but also various services offered in the hospitals. Patient satisfaction measurement adds important information in terms of system performance, thus contributing to the organisation's total quality management. The study is necessated because decease burden is increasing day by day as shown in Figure 3.

QoL is considered to be the vital health outcome measure for cancer patients' care. It is a term integrating various aspects of life such as physical, psychological, socio-economical, spiritual, cognitive, and social dimensions. It is also defined as the present lifestyle, past experiences, future hopes, dreams, and ambitions.

A good QoL can lead to better longevity of life in cancer patients. This aspect has remained neglected in the medical field, and it's high time now that the research should stress the importance of QoL in increasing longevity of life in cancer patients. With this background, the present study aims to fulfil the following objectives, discussed next.

1.2 Objectives

1. To identify the determinants in QoL for cancer patients
2. To measure association between QoL and survival of cancer patients
3. To suggest improvement in behaviour change and communication recommendations for improving life standards

1.3 Justification of the Work

The measurement of the QoL index assessment can assist with decision making and provide data in clinical trials and identify patients who need psychosocial interventions. As the diagnosis and management of cancer can have a major impact on every aspect of a patient's QoL, this may help many patients to increase their well-being. Despite its importance, QoL is rarely a reported outcome in randomised clinical trials in cancer patients; failure to collect data on QoL may reflect a lack of information among researchers and clinicians about the adequacy and relative merits of the measures available for assessing it. This small study will be a driving force to initiate and develop methodologies and steps to ameliorate the conditions of cancer patients.

CHAPTER 2

Review of Literature

2.1 Review of Literature

Quality of life (QoL) is a multidimensional concept that includes quite a few features of life such as physical health status, psychological well-being, and people's emotional, social, and cognitive functions, along with its impact on disease and treatment on patients' lives. When the individual well-being is fulfilled as per these expectations, standards, and concerns, than we say the patient has a decent QoL, and it might be expressed in terms of satisfaction, happiness, pleasure, and accomplishment. QoL parameters must take into account all types of treatment whether physical or mental so that they may help in selecting more suitable treatment options. Several studies have been conducted to assess the QoL worldwide but are limited in India. A few important contributions are cited next.

Patiño et al. (2005) evaluated patients before the intervention and later on after 1, 3, and 6 months. QoL and nutritional status remained stable in most of the patients the study reported on.

Santangelo et al. (2006) concluded that terminally ill oncological patients are treatable with palliative cures, representing a treatment system aimed at improving the QoL of both the patient and the family members, decreasing the physical and psychical suffering of the patient.

DOI: 10.1201/9781003437994-2

Echteld et al. (2007) studied the changes in individual quality of life (I-QoL) and its associations in patients admitted to a palliative care unit. The results show that mean I-QoL scores improved notably. A high correlation was found between I-QoL and the relationships with family members and friends.

Saad et al. (2007) investigated the predictors of QoL improvement among patients undergoing parenchyma resection due to lung cancer. Thirty-six patients with lung cancer diagnosis were assessed before surgery. Anxiety and depressive symptoms might be among factors affecting the QoL after lung cancer surgery; therefore screening and treatment of these symptoms might help to improve QoL in this group.

Madhusudhan et al. (2009) assessed QoL after palliative stenting in patients with inoperable oesophageal cancer. The use of a self-expanding metal stent (SEMS) is a well-established modality for palliation of dysphagia in such patients. The global health status and all functional scores improved significantly after stenting from baseline until 8 weeks. This shows that use of SEMS resulted in significant improvement in all scales of QoL without any mortality and acceptable morbidity.

Dehkordi et al. (2009) conducted a study on QoL in cancer patients undergoing chemotherapy and suffering from tumours which were solid in nature and were subjected to varying chemotherapy dosages and cycles. They recommended that cancer patients be encouraged to complete a chemotherapy (CT) course which plays a significant role in the treatment and its outcome. It also helps the QoL in cancer patients undergoing CT to achieve better outcomes. In 2011, the authors replicated the study, and the outcomes were found to be similar.

Dubashi et al. (2010) reported that overall QoL in breast cancer patients who are in an early stage of their life appeared good on average. The breast conservation group was compared with the mastectomy group, and the QoL and sexual function were marginally worse in mastectomy group. Cervical cancer was the most common type of cancer, and it is reported to be the main cause of death in Indian women, and it also affects the QoL.

Kannan et al. (2011) assessed the QoL of cancer patients with the use of a validated questionnaire, and 11 different types of cancer were chosen. They reported that among the total respondents, 80% of them have average or below-average QoL. The findings suggest that there is growing importance that must be given to the incorporation of QoL treatment in addition to other clinical endpoints.

Elsaie et al. (2012) conducted a study on most functional magnitudes of QoL for colorectal cancer patients. The study found all symptoms decreased except fatigue, and there was noticeable reduction in physical, role, and cognitive functioning, as well as overall functioning following the chemotherapy session. QoL and number of treatment cycles were found highly related. Various other cancer-related factors are also supposed to affect the QoL. Among women, breast cancer was the most frequently occurring cancer, and it is ranked third among all cancer-related deaths.

D'Souza et al. (2013) conducted a study in head and neck cancer (HNC) patients to assess the QoL and its performance status. To find an association between QoL, demographic and disease variables were identified. The Karnofsky Performance Status (KPS) scale was adopted to assess the performance status. Subjects with all stages of HNC and primarily diagnosed cancers were used in the study. The findings concluded that among patients with HNC, physical, psychological, social, spiritual, and other functional domains are affected.

Akça et al. (2014) evaluated the changes in QoL among breast cancer patients who had undergone surgical treatment. Patients treated with breast-preserving surgery (BPS), modified radical mastectomy (MRM), and simple mastectomy (SM) in different age groups were taken into account. Turkish versions of the EORTC QLQ-C30 and

EORTC–BR23 questionnaires, which are well validated, were used for the study. The MRM group was found to be more adversely affected than the BPS group as reported by the study.

Using a sample of 280 patients, Hemavathy and Julius (2016) conducted a study to explore the QoL among women with cervical cancer. Among cervical cancer patients, QoL was found to be a very crucial aspect in developing countries, including India. There is a strong need to assess the QoL among such patients and relevant measures to cervical cancer survivors for their better treatment and enhanced QoL.

One domain area of well-being has significant effects on the other related domains of QoL, and there is a strong relationship between the performance status and QoL as well. Despite the best information available at my disposal, limited studies are available on the QoL in different types of cancer in India, and those available are mainly specific to breast cancer. Cancer the disease and its treatment could lead to different types of changes in the life of the patient, which could be the general well-being or physical, psychological, and social status of the patient. Findings from various studies show that there is no visible correlation between the QoL and age, sex, marital status, educational status, duration of disease, economic condition, and occupational functions of the cancer patient. The problem in the case of long-term survivors with respect to social or emotional support, spiritual and philosophical views of life, and health status was also prominent. Measures should be taken to diminish the gap between expectation and reality so that a greater satisfaction could be realised among cancer patients and thus an improved QoL.

Thus we see that very few studies are done in this direction, and the present study will be a small step towards recommended small changes for improving QoL of cancer patients.

CHAPTER 3

Background of Study Area

The Indian health care industry is growing at a slow pace with a growth rate of 13% annually. The Indian middle class is seeking a better quality of health care services and thus driving the demand for quality health care. The continuous expansion of private hospitals and increased spending on health could raise the growth rate further. Factors that could drive the overall demand and thus growth include an ageing population, growing urbanisation, higher awareness, more skilled professionals, low-cost treatments, improved infrastructure, health insurance, telemedicine, Business Process Outsourcing (BPOs), and health tourism.

Tertiary care is generally associated with the health care facilities provided at specialty and super specialty hospitals. These hospitals also act as training centres for doctors and other allied health care–related workforces. These institutions are mainly equipped with ultra-modern equipment, the knowledge of whose working provides the trainee with the advanced and updated hands-on experience with the latest technologies. During the last few years, there has been a sudden increase in the occurrence of cancer and related diseases, both communicable and non-communicable.

In the case of any medical or surgical emergencies, including those caused due to causalities, the patient is

DOI: 10.1201/9781003437994-3

13

usually referred to the nearest city hospital after first-aid treatment being provided. In very serious cases, the patient is further advised to go to big cities for treatment, without taking into consideration the financial condition of the family. For better management of the disease and welfare of the patients, often they are further referred to speciality care units within the city. But the problem is enhanced even more, when these super specialty hospitals, being the last hope for the poor and helpless families, are themselves ill and mismanaged. In most of the cases, these super hospitals turn out to be of no benefit for the common man at the time when help is highly need. All this happens because of an unofficial parallel dual system of health care delivery in India. The kind of services people are entitled to depends upon their economic status, which is a big concern.

With regard to resource allocation, secondary and tertiary care suffer the most. This is due to the expansion of tertiary health care facilities, needs, and considerable resources to adequately respond to the needs of state-of-the-art diagnostic procedures and treatment complexities. Most state government budgets meet the recurrent costs to maintain existing levels of public health care, which is a major component of budgetary allocations. In most states of the country, salaries and wages account for around 70% of the total health budget, scarcely leaving any resources for expansion of services. Tertiary care services are relatively more expensive as compared to primary or secondary care services, and their establishment and maintenance are big issues. As a result, such services in the public sector are limited, given the total expenditure on public health out of gross domestic product (GDP). As a result, the availability of tertiary care services is skewed towards the private domain vis-à-vis the public sector, and the associated costs again drive the private sector to get concentrated in urban areas. Geographical inequities are also clearly visible in this case. Tertiary care health services in India are concentrated towards big cities, and there is a gross inequity between rural and urban setups. People in rural areas seeking such services are forced to travel to the big cities. More often than not, they need to go to the major metropolitan cities as well to get the necessary treatments. Lack of advanced infrastructure in the rural areas is to a large extent because of the lack of trained manpower in the field. There are various other problems faced by rural patients like overcrowding, delayed consultation, lack of proper guidance, etc., which lead to patient dissatisfaction. Today patients are looking for hassle-free and quick services. This could be possible only with optimum utility of the scarce resources through a multitasking scenario in Outpatient Department (OPD) for better, efficient, and effective services. The brief description of the three hospitals included in the study is given next.

3.1 King George's Medical University (KGMU)

The KGMU was built in 1905, and it has acquired national and global eminence for its contributions in academics, medical research, and patient care. The first batch of MBBS students entered the portals of the erstwhile KGMC in October 1911, and 31 doctors passed in the year 1916. Since then, KGMC has produced over 20,000 alumni who are serving in India and all over the world. The college was given a status of university in 2002 by a special Act of the Government of Uttar Pradesh. It is now the largest residential medical university in India with 48 buildings and 80 teaching departments in four faculties (Medical, Dental, Paramedical, and Nursing). An 'A' grade certification has been awarded to KGMU by the National Assessment and Accreditation Council (NAAC), which will remain valid from May 2017 to May 2022 and 'A+' rating at present in 2023.

The separate Division of Oncology was established in the Surgery Department of KGMU, Lucknow, in the year 1979 by the government of Uttar Pradesh (UP). Prof. NC Misra headed this unit for the next 17 years, and under his guidance the Oncology Department established itself as a premier centre for excellence in academics, research, and training with clinical services relating to different types of cancer.

Over the years, the Oncology Division has carried the major responsibility for providing tertiary care for cancer patients from UP, neighbouring states, and Nepal. The Department of Surgical Oncology is functioning in the newly established Shatabdi Phase I and II buildings. One exclusive floor of the Shatabdi Phase building holds the administrative offices, consultants' rooms, library, seminar hall, records, in-patient wards, and day care with CT facilities. Postoperative wards along with four modular operation theatres are located on the second floor of the Shatabdi Phase I building. The two buildings of the Shatabdi hospitals are connected by a bridge on the second floor.

According to an annual report (2016):

Bed Strength:	The average bed occupancy rate is 98–100%.
Annual OPD attendance:	26,153
Annual indoor admissions:	3605
Annual chemotherapies administered:	7978
Annual major/minor operations:	1977

The Department of Radiotherapy was created on 16 December 1986 when the Radiology Department was split into two distinct Departments of Radiotherapy and Radio-diagnosis. The original department (Integrated Department of Radiology) was established in the year 1927 at this college. Many courses such as diploma in medical radiology and electrology (DMRE) were started from 1940 and MD (Radiology) since 1953. Radiotherapy and associated treatments were started with two deep therapy x-ray units in the 1950s. A superficial therapy unit (Maximar:100) came into existence in 1960, and the first cobalt unit (Gammatron: II) in 1963. After the split of the Integrated Department of Radiology, Prof. G N Agarwal became its first head for only the 'Department of Radiotherapy'. A new cobalt unit (Theratron:780 C) along with a treatment simulator (Shimadzu SAT: 10) was installed in 1989. Treatment planning systems (TSG: Radplan) and an ultrasound machine (Wipro GE RT: 3200) were installed in 1994 and 1999, correspondingly. A new cobalt unit (Theratron: 780 E) was installed in the year 2004. A Plato Planning and Oncentra Contouring System was added in the department in the year 2005. Initiation of a high-dose rate brachytherapy (HDR: BT) unit was done in the year 2008. A radiotherapy simulator (Simulix Evolution and Nucletron) was installed in the year 2009. An indigenous cobalt unit (Bhabhatron- II) was donated to the department by Atomic Energy, Government of India in 2010. A new 16-slice wide-bore CT simulator, was installed in the year 2013. A new linear accelerator (Elekta-Synergy) has been fixed in the department which is under the commissioning process at present. At present the department offers six seats annually for the MD (Radiotherapy) course and three seats for senior residents in the dept. The department offers OPD services at all working days. It has 65 beds strength for indoor patient and 16 beds in the day care unit. Clinical services provided include radiotherapy (comprising external beam radiotherapy and also brachytherapy), chemotherapy, and a CT simulator.

Recent additions in the department include the following:

1. Colour Doppler facility (since 2002)
2. 3D-TPS planning (since 2005)
3. Telemedicine facility from 2007 in collaboration with the Department of Radiotherapy, SGPGI, Lucknow
4. HDR-BT unit (since 2008)

5. Radiotherapy simulator unit (since 2009)
6. One Bhabhatron unit (since 2010)
7. Endoscopy facility (since 2010)
8. Bronchoscope facility (since 2010)
9. Photodynamic therapy (since 2011)
10. 16-slice wide-bore CT simulator (since 2013)
11. High energy linear accelerator (process of commissioning)

For future planning, KGMU is trying to build a comprehensive cancer institute, and the proposal for the same has been sent to the government of UP for perusal.

3.2 Sanjay Gandhi Postgraduate Institute of Medical Sciences (SGPGIMS)

SGPGIMS, Lucknow, India, is an institute established under State Act, 1983. The institute is located on a 550-acre residential campus at Raebareli Road, 15 km away from the main city of Lucknow. SGPGIMS offers its own degrees in medical science, duly recognised by the Medical Council of India. The institute is top rated amongst the medical institutes in the country, bringing state-of-the-art tertiary medical care facilities, super-specialty teaching, advanced training, and researches. The dedicated faculty works hard to provide quality education, patient care, and research. The institute endeavours to meet the challenges and requirements of the society as needed. The institute offers DM, MCh, MD, and PhD degrees; postdoctoral fellowships (PDFs); postdoctoral certificate courses (PDCCs); and senior residencies in several specialties. The peers in the field have acknowledged the courses offered by the institution. Candidates obtaining degrees from SGPGIMS are placed high both within and outside of the country.

SGPGI, Lucknow, is a referral hospital, and patients are asked to bring a note from the referring doctor or hospital in which they were treated. The physicians who refer are requested to mention the nature of disease, the specialty they require from the referred institute for the patient, and the nature of support required from the institute. The institute referred works on an appointment system of its own. The patients are then advised to revisit the hospital only on the appointed days, except in case of an emergency. All facilities at the hospital are available on a self-financed basis, and there is hardly any provision for free treatment or diagnosis. The institute relies totally on its own blood bank for blood requirements and expects the patients' families or friends to provide replacement blood. The institute caters to all emergencies services related to the specialties present at the hospital. As the hospital does not possess all specialties, it does not cater to general medical emergencies at present. If the disease does not relate to the specialties at the institution, they are given only the basic first aid and then referred to other institutions.

3.2.1 Department of Radiotherapy

The Department of Radiotherapy was established to deliver quality-oriented, state-of-the art, complete radiotherapy care to all such facilities that do not exist in the state of UP or its surrounding areas. The building plan was approved by the Bhabha Atomic Research Centre (BARC), Mumbai, and the foundation stone of this department was laid on 17 August 1988. In the beginning only two faculty members were recruited i.e., in October 1987.

The construction of the department was finished in a short span of 2 years, and it became functional since August 1990. It was expected to create the basic infrastructure which includes the buildings, obtaining of equipment, and their installation within this short period of time. After getting the necessary clearance from BARC, Mumbai, on 7 August 1990, the first patient was treated on the telecobalt unit—the Theratron-780C. From then, the department has been enthusiastically involved in tracking its goal towards providing quality health care in radiation-oncology for patients who are referred both from within SGPGI and those referred from other medical colleges/hospitals from UP and the neighbouring states.

Currently around 60% of the patients registered at the hospital come from the super-specialties of the hospital, and the rest are referred cases from other hospitals. Head and neck, gastrointestinal, gynaecological, urological, breast, and central nervous system malignancies are the most common cancers that are being treated in this department. Out-patient services are operative only for 5 days a week i.e., Monday to Friday.

The departmental motto is 'Quality assured radiation therapy'. The department is well prepared in all aspects, including equipment and trained manpower. With an extremely devoted and motivated team of doctors, the institute constantly is on the path of achieving its goal. It is furnished with up-to-date facilities including a dual-energy linear accelerator, HDR-BT systems, telecobalt unit, simulators, computerised 3-D radiation therapy planning systems, and mould room facilities for the fabrication of blocks, compensators, and other devices to facilitate a smooth flow of work. Also, there is a physics laboratory to provide the backup maintenance to deliver and monitor quality radiation therapy for the cancer patients. The department started interstitial HDR-BT when the installation of the HDR-Microselectron commenced in August 1997. Later with the installation of the new simulator CT and ISIS 3-D treatment planning system in 2002, the efficiency increased. The TSG Radplan treatment planning system was elevated in January 2005.

The institution has been bestowed a position of as Regional Cancer Care Centre by the Ministry of Health and Family Welfare for the strength of its present cancer treatment services by the proposal sent to the Department of Radiotherapy. A grant of Rs 50 million was released to enlarge the cancer treatment facilities. The department, when enlarged, will be able to deal with the facilities for stereotactic radiotherapy and radiosurgery, conformational therapy, online portal imaging facilities, and image-guided radiotherapy.

The department of Endocrine and Breast Surgery at SGPGIMS, Lucknow, has been a pioneer in the field of clinical practices, training, and teaching along with conducting research in various areas of endocrine and breast surgery in UP and India. Established in September 1989, this was the first academic department of endocrine and breast surgery in the nation that offers an opportunity for devoted training in a related specialty. The PDCC in endocrine surgery was first stated in India in 1997 at this department, and was later one of the first to start a 3-year MCh Endocrine Surgery course in the year 2004 after obtaining the necessary permissions from the Medical Council of India (MCI). Further, it has six faculty members and the sanctioned strength of four MCh students every year. Hospital services, senior residents, and short-term trainees from time to time also work, besides having research staff, technicians, and other office staff. Distinguished alumni of the department are currently involved in academic practices and medical treatment practice for endocrine and breast surgery in several parts of India and abroad. They are mostly professors, heads, faculty members, or senior consultants in numerous esteemed teaching organisations or corporate hospitals in all the foremost cities of the nation.

The department receives an enormous number of referrals from several parts of India and neighbouring countries (mainly Nepal) for complex endocrine and breast surgical treatments, and is recognised as one of the few high-quality centres for complex repeat thyroid surgery, primary hyperparathyroidism surgery, pheochromocytoma and other adrenal tumours, and breast conservation and oncoplastic surgical procedures. It is also considered part of comprehensive multimodal treatment for early and advanced breast cancers with high precision. The department has established minimally invasive endocrine surgical procedures, particularly laparoscopic adrenal surgery, minimally invasive parathyroidectomy, and video-assisted thoracoscopic thymectomy and sentinel lymph node biopsy along with conservation/oncoplastic breast surgery. The department and faculty members have effectively carried out and are presently engaged in devoted clinical as well as basic research in the field of endocrine oncology.

3.3 Ram Manohar Lohia Hospital (RML)

The Dr Ram Manohar Lohia Institute of Medical Sciences (RMLIMS) is an autonomous, multispeciality medical institute established by the government of UP. The chairperson is Mr Anup Chandra Pandey, chief secretary, government of Uttar Pradesh. The vice chairperson of the institute is Dr Rajneesh Dube, principal secretary. The institution is located in Vibhuti Khand, Gomti Nagar, Lucknow. The hospital affiliated with the institute offers high-end and excellent facilities and the best treatments in several super-speciality medical areas. The institution also deals with teaching services, imparting degrees in DM, MCh, MD, MS, and PhD along with giving diplomas in paramedical programmes.

The hospital functions as a referral centre for the enormous population of Lucknow and also of the adjacent districts catering to the eastern belt of UP. Services are stretched to all sections of society, particularly for the poor and downtrodden population of the region who require specialised care. The hospital provides inclusive care for cancer patients with well-developed amenities and proficiency in surgical procedures, radiation, and medical and laboratory oncology along with nuclear medicine. Specialities in cardiology, cardiothoracic surgery, gastrointestinal medicine, gastro-surgery, nephrology, urology, neurology, and neurosurgery are also well established at this hospital. Speciality clinics including refractory epilepsy, pain clinic, uro-oncology, dialysis, lithotripsy, and a catheterisation lab, are functional along with a well-built intensive care unit (ICU).

The institution offers state-of-the-art diagnostic facilities in health care. The Department of Pathology and Microbiology has been elevated to a 'State Referral Centre for Laboratory Investigations'. The Department of Radiology has developed high-end services with an inclusive 64-slice CT scan, three Tesla MRI machines, bone mineral density (BMD), mammography, etc., along with interventional radiology services. The hospital is networked by an all-inclusive web-based hospital information system (HIS) that offers electronic records from registration to discharge of the patients. Online registration, bidirectional web-based lab reporting, picture archiving and communication system (PACS) system for image transfer, e-pharmacy, and webmail are also available here. The faculty of the institution comprises keen and skilled doctors showing devotion towards growth and development in health care and patient well-being. The administrative hierarchy comprises the director, finance controller, engineers, and joint director material management.

CHAPTER **4**

Methodology

4.1 Conceptual Framework

The Life Quality Index (LQI) is a compound social indicator for assessing human welfare that reflects the expected length of life, good health, and improvement of the quality of life (QoL) through access to income. The LQI combines two primary social indicators: the expectancy of a healthy life at birth and the real gross domestic product per person, corrected with purchasing power parity as needed. Both are widely obtainable and precise statistics for QoL. QoL research is especially important in the area of cancer survivorship, not only because there are so many survivors but also because most patients receive some form of adjuvant therapy in addition to surgery and because of the increasing timelines for certain therapies lasting for years. In addition, the long natural history of the disease makes treatment outcomes uncertain as to whether a patient is ever cured. Psychosocial complications multiply the hardships of physical symptoms along with affecting the QoL of cancer patients. The psychosocial suffering that the patients feel upon diagnosis may upset their treatment because these symptoms can be irresistible.

DOI: 10.1201/9781003437994-4

4.2 Hypothesis

1. H_{01}: The QoL index has no correlation with age
2. H_{02}: Factors affecting QoL are associated with patient well-being

Uttar Pradesh (UP) is chosen as a research area because, on the one hand, it has the highest population density and, on the other hand, its health development indicators are poor. There is an urgent need for intervention in this geographical area, as it has a very high number of cancer patients with poor treatment facilities. Moreover, the majority of patients have financial constraints which accelerate their stress and further deteriorate their health. It will be a cross-sectional study by collecting data from three oncology centres in Lucknow. Lucknow is the capital city of UP and treats almost 90% of the severely suffering cancer patients at the advanced stage of the disease in UP at some point of their treatment. All the patients attending oncology centres both in OPD (OPD means coming to the hospital and consulting with a doctor and going back home without being admitted) and indoors (indoor patient means those who are admitted in the hospital for treatment) were included in the study, who agreed to participate and gave written consent. Patients who were suffering in last stage or with other complications and didn't give consent could be excluded from the study. Ethical clearance was taken from institutional ethical committees. History and findings of clinical examination, including mobility, history of discharge, retraction, etc., were noted.

4.3 Sampling Framework

It was found that around 5000 cancer patients visit King Goerge's Medical College (KGMC) annually as per the record register. The picture is not much different in Sanjay Gandhi Postgraduate Institute of Medical Sciences (SGPGI), but in Ram Manohar Lohia (RML), as it is new, the footfall (footfall means less number of patients as compared to other 2 hospitals) is less. RML has its own oncology department furnished with all modern infrastructure facilities and high-tech equipment. Non-probability purposive sampling was done. The sample of about 300 patients from three tertiary care units were collected based on the sample size assessment as follows:

$$N = Z^2 P(1-P)/e^2$$

Where:

N is the total sample size required
Z value is taken at 95% confidence interval (1.96)
P is the 60% prevalence as per record 2012 of ICMR
e is 1% of the probable error
$(1.96)^2 (0.6) (0.4)/(0.1)^2$
$= 92.19 \sim 100$

Hence we sampled more than 100 patients from each hospital with the help of the OPD doctor on duty, leading to the final sample of 310. We tried to select the patient on the day of visit who had been diagnosed with any type of cancer and at any stage of cancer but had started treatment. The same patients were followed for 6 months, as we took their appointment dates to follow them. Also the help of the patient registry system was used for the follow-up. As some patients did not turn up within the period of 6 months, they could not be sampled; the reason for not turning up could not be traced, and as a result there was a reduction in follow-up cases.

Patients were followed after 6 months to assess the change in QoL after the interventions of doctor and treatment.

4.4 Tools and Technique Used

QoL was measured using Ferrell's QoL questionnaire. Ferrell summarised the definitions of the four QoL domains:

- Physical well-being is the control or relief of symptoms and the maintenance of function and independence.
- Psychological well-being is the attempt to maintain a sense of control in the face of life-threatening illness characterised by emotional distress, altered life priorities, and fear of the unknown, as well as positive life changes.
- Social well-being is the effort to deal with the impact of cancer on individuals, their roles, and relationships.
- Spiritual well-being is the ability to maintain hope and derive meaning from the cancer experience, which is characterised by uncertainty.

The EORTC Quality of Life questionnaire is a 46-item inventory that enables patients to evaluate QoL on a scale of 0 to 10, where 0 indicates the worst QoL and 10 the best. The scale evaluates general QoL, psychological well-being, distress owing to illness and treatment, fearfulness, social concerns, and spiritual well-being. An attempt will be made to evaluate the change in overall QoL and change in QoL for different dimensions.

QoL: This was measured by summing all the scores of 46 items and then the index was built by using the following formula:

$$QoL = \frac{Actual\ score}{Maximum\ Theoretical\ Score}$$

Here the highest score is 460, as there are 46 items rated on the scale of 0–10.

4.5 Confirmatory Factor Analysis (CFA)

The next step was to conduct CFA. This is a type of structural equation modelling (SEM) that deals explicitly with measurement models, which suggest the relationships between observed measures or indicators and latent variables or factors (Brown, 2006). Here the set of theoretical relationships among measured variables and their respective latent constructs are tested. Furthermore, the CFA procedure needs to be performed simultaneously for all latent constructs. The measurement model could be assessing based on unidimensionality, validity, and reliability. Unidimensionality can be achieved when measuring items have acceptable factor loading for the individual latent construct. Factor loadings lower than 0.6 should be deleted from the latent constructs in the model to ensure unidimensionality is satisfied (Brown, 2006; Mohd Zainudin et al., 2012). If all the factor loadings are greater than 0.6, unidimensionality for the model has been achieved. The redundant or correlated items in the model should be examined through the Modification Index (MI). An MI higher than 15 indicates that the items correlated. So the items will be deleted or set as free parameters to achieve the fitness of the model. This was done for all five constructs of the data.

4.6 Structural Equation Modelling

SEM was developed as a unifying and flexible mathematical framework to specify the computer application (Byrne, 2001; Blunch, 2012). The two main components of SEM are the structural model and the measurement model. The path model or path analysis developed by Sewall (1923) quantifies specific cause-and-effect relationships between observed variables and was later pioneered by (Bollen, 1989; Jöreskog, 1993). The measurement model quantifies linkages between:

1. Hypothetical constructs that might be known but unobservable components

2. Observed variables that represent a specific hypothetical construct in the form of a linear combination

Given that SEM is profoundly filled with jargon, mainly
regarding the types of variables hypothesised in the model,
an introductory definition of terms will allow for a clearer
description of the findings. Some of the common termi-
nologies used in SEM include:

- *Exogenous Variables*—Variables which are not
  influenced by other variables in the defined model.
- *Endogenous Variables*—Variables which are influenced by other variables in the defined model.
- *Indicator Variables*—Variables which are directly
  observed and measured.
- *Latent Variables*—Variables which are not directly
  measured in the model.
- *Measurement Model*—This is the main part of the
  full structural equation model diagram hypothesised for the study, and it includes all observations
  that load onto the latent variables, their relationships, variances, and errors.
- *Structural Model*—This is also part of the total
  hypothesised structural equation model diagram, and
  this comprises both latent and indicator variables.
- *Structural Equation Model*—This model combines
  the structural model and the measurement model
  and comprises everything that has been measured or observed between the variables that are
  examined.

The SEM allows the addition of latent variables into the
analyses, and it is not limited only to relationship measurement between observed variables and constructs.
Rather, it allows the study to measure any combinations
of relationships through exploring a series of dependent
relationships concurrently, while considering potential
errors of measurement between all variables. SEM has
numerous advantages over conventional analysis. This

includes greater flexibility about assumptions (even in the face of multicollinearity, it allows interpretation). SEM allows the use of CFA to decrease measurement error by testing multiple indicators per latent variable, along with offering superior model visualisation through its graphical modelling interface (Hatcher, 2005; Jöreskog, 1993; Kline, 2005). Moreover, SEM has the interesting ability of testing models overall rather than coefficients individually. It also has the capability to test models with multiple dependent variables that include mediating variables to the model error terms for all indicator variables also.

The overall structural equation model structure can be distilled into three matrix equations: Two for the measurement model component and the remaining one for the structural model component (Grace, 2006).

The measurement model for exogenous (x) and endogenous (y) latent variables can be written as:

$$x = \lambda \xi + \delta \qquad (1)$$

$$y = \gamma \eta + \varepsilon \qquad (2)$$

Where:

x is an observed exogenous variable
ξ is an exogenous latent variable
δ is a measurement error
λ is a factor loading relating $\mathbf{x}$ to ξ
y is an observed endogenous variable
η is an endogenous latent variable
ε is a measurement error for the observed endogenous variables
γ is a factor loading relating y to η

The structural model component as relationships among latent construct variables can be written as:

$$\eta = \beta \eta + \Gamma \xi + \zeta \qquad (3)$$

Where β is a path coefficient describing the relationships among endogenous latent variables.

Γ is a path coefficient describing the linear effects of exogenous variables on endogenous variables
ζ is errors of endogenous variables

For the estimation process, most SEM computer programmes and most structural equation models are estimated by using the maximum likelihood estimated method. Amos 21 was used for the analysis purpose along with SPSS.

Chapter 5

Data Analysis

5.1 Data Analysis

A cross-sectional study was conducted in three tertiary care hospitals in Lucknow. The respondents were sampled from these hospitals, viz; KGMU, SGPGIMS, and RMLIMS. These super-speciality hospitals with modern infrastructure facilities are situated in Lucknow only; hence, people from all over the state along with adjoining states like Bihar Jharkhand Chhattisgarh, etc., are referred to these places. The city also caters to a few private hospitals but the majority of the population still prefers these hospitals for cancer treatment due to their skilled doctors.

Patients with cancer of various types and belonging to various regions of Uttar Pradesh (UP) attending the departments of oncology, gynaecology, radiology, etc., were included. Patients received chemotherapy as both an in-patient and an out-patient.

5.2 Data

The questionnaires consist of five parts along with respondents' general profiles. It contains five function subscales (physical well-being, psychological well-being, fear, social well-being, spiritual well-being). The Quality of Life Instrument with a 46-item ordinal scale (0–9) was

DOI: 10.1201/9781003437994-5

used to measure the quality of life of a cancer patient. This tool has proven to be useful in clinical practice along with research. The scoring was based on a scale of 0 as the worst outcome to 10 as the best outcome. Several items have reverse anchors and therefore were coded by reversing the scores of those items.

There are five latent exogenous constructs, namely physical well-being (F1), psychological well-being (F2), fear (F3), social well-being (F4), spiritual well-being (F5), and one endogenous construct which is quality of life (QoL).

The **F1** construct is measured by nine items, which are fatigue (R1), appetite change (R2), pain (R3), sleep change (R4), weight change (R5), constipation (R6), nausea (R7), menstrual change (R8), and overall physical health (G9).

The **F2** construct is measured by 17 items, which are difficulty in coping with the disease (R10), difficulty in coping with treatment (R11), deterioration in QoL (R12), feeling of unhappiness (R13), lack of control (Psy14), unsatisfied with life (Psy15), loss of memory (Psy16), non-usefulness (Psy17), appearance change (R18), self-concept change (Psy19), initial diagnosis problem (R20), chemotherapy problem (R21), radiation problem (R22), surgery problem (R23), post-treatment problem (R24), anxiety (R25), and depression (R26).

The **F3** construct is measured by five items, which are fear of future tests (R27), second cancer (R28), recurrence (R29), spreading (R30), and feeling normal (Fr31).

The **F4** construct is measured by eight items, which are distress for family (Soc32), family support (Soc33), personal relationship (R34), sex life (R35), job (R36), household activities (R37), isolation (R38), and financial burden (R39).

The **F5** construct is measured by seven items, which are religious activities (Spr40), meditation (Spr41), spiritual change (Spr42), uncertainty (R43), positive change (Spr44), purpose of life (Spr45), and hope (Spr46).

The QoL for cancer patients is observed using physical well-being (F1), psychological well-being (F2), fear (F3), social well-being (F4), and spiritual well-being (F5). This report tries to study the relationship between these observed variables and QoL.

5.2.1 General Profile

Most of the respondents were from a rural background, and Lucknow is the capital city, most of the tertiary care government hospitals with the most modern infrastructure and highly qualified doctors are found there, and above all, people from almost the entire state are referred to these hospitals for advanced treatment. Purposive sampling was done to cater to the total sample of 310 respondents. As nearly two-thirds of the UP population lives in rural areas, we see that the sample is the true representation of the population with reference to living location.

As we see from Figure 4, the majority of the population belongs to rural areas with low socio-economic status (Figure 5). Nearly 71.8% of the population belongs to a lower-income group with a very low standard of living. This is also one of the major reasons that they are more

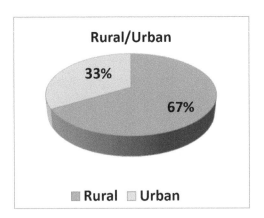

FIGURE 4 Distribution of respondents (age-wise).

Source: Srivastava, Tiwari et al., 2019.

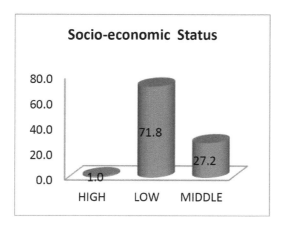

FIGURE 5   Bar plot of patients' socioeconomic status.

Source: Srivastava, Tiwari et al., 2019.

vulnerable to health hazards. Due to a lack of money they cannot afford the right treatment at the right time and at the right place (hospital). By the time they really get the right diagnosis, treatment is delayed which further aggravates their problems.

Another important factor is awareness level that largely depends upon the literacy level. After so many initiatives by the government the illiteracy level was recorded as high, nearly 27%. Only 17.3% of the respondents were graduate level and 5.8% were post-graduate level. This is one of the major hurdles in achieving a better QoL even without disease, and those with a disease like cancer lead a worse life.

As we see from Figure 6, the respondents are basically from the rural or low-income background, so the educational status is also low.

With respect to gender distribution as seen in Figure 7, it has been observed that the female accounts a little higher than the male in the sampled population. The main reason could be the prevalence of breast cancer, which is quite high in India.

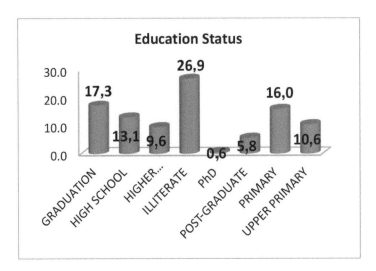

FIGURE 6 Bar plot of education level among cancer patients.

Mostly the respondents were married, with only 7% unmarried and 4% were widowed or divorced as seen in Figure 8. The main reason is that elderly people are more prone to cancer than children or adolescents.

Table 1 shows the occupational status of the respondents. As more than half of the respondents are female, the majority are housewives. The respondents show a low

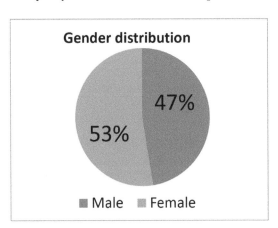

FIGURE 7 Pie chart of gender distribution.

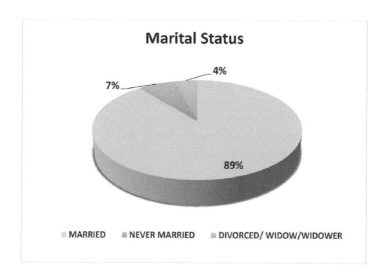

FIGURE 8 Pie chart of marital status.

income because 9.3% are farmers and 7.7% are labourers. Also 3.3% of respondents were students with no income and 2.2% retired with no or marginal income. Government employee/professional were only 15.7% and self-employed account for 13.1%.

TABLE 1 Occupational Status

Occupation	Percentage
Farmer	9.3
Govt. Employee/Professionals	15.7
Housewife	39.1
Labourer	9.6
Retired	2.2
Self-Employed	13.1
Student	3.2
Unemployed	7.7
Total	100.0

5.2.2 Age Distribution

The age of the patient varies from 12 to 81 years, covering almost all age groups except infants. Out of a total 312 respondents, we have only 5 patients below 18 years of age. The maximum of patients suffering from cancer lies between 36 and 55 years of age i.e., nearly 53% of the patients are in middle-age group. Almost all the cases in this age group are diagnosed within a year and treatment started after some time except one case which was diagnosed 3 years back but treatment started after the lapse of 34 months as seen in Table 2.

But in the age group 46–55 we have many cases in which there is a lapse in the time of treatment and diagnosis by more than a year. In two extreme cases of uterine cancer, it was diagnosed 5–6 years back, but treatment started after the lapse of 5 years.

5.2.3 Body Mass Index (BMI)

The BMI status of 31.7% of the respondents was normal i.e. it ranges from 20.0 to 24.9, and nearly 17.3% lie below normal as seen in Table 3. We see a high percentage of the population suffering from obesity of degree I. There are 7.4% of respondents who are over obese, and it is a matter of concern. On the other hand we see that respondents are

TABLE 2   Age Distribution

S. No.	Age Group	Percentage (n)
1	12–17	1.60 (5)
2	18–25	6.41 (20)
3	26–35	17.95 (56)
4	36–45	27.24 (85)
5	46–55	25.96 (81)
6	56–65	15.38 (48)
7	66–75	4.17 (13)
8	76–85	1.28 (4)

TABLE 3   Obesity (grading as per James et al., 1988)

BMI	Nutritional Grade	Percentage of Cases (n = 312)
<16.00	Malnourished (III degree)	6.1(19)
16.0–16.9	Malnourished (II degree)	4.5(14)
17.0–17.9	Malnourished (I degree)	6.1(19)
18.0–19.9	Low normal	17.3(54)
20.0–24.9	Normal	31.7(99)
25.0–30.0	Overweight (I degree obese)	26.9(84)
>30.0	Over obese	7.4(23)

also suffering from malnourishment of grade I, II, and III and belong to the age group of 18–65 years.

5.2.4 Type of Cancer

It was seen that 25.6% of patients suffer from oral cancer followed by 25% of patients (women) suffering from breast cancer as shown in Table 4. This finding is also supported by the finding of the National Institute of Cancer Prevention and Research (NICPR) where the maximum number of cases is reported from oral and breast cancer in India. Other types of cancers through which patients are majorly affected are gastrointestinal 9.6%, uterus 9%, and respiratory 9.6%. Patients suffering from blood, prostate, and ear cancers are very negligible, at nearly 0.3%. Endocrine, colon, bone, and skin cancer also affect around 3–4% of the population.

5.2.5 Diagnosis and Treatment

Regarding the time of diagnosis, it was seen that in most of the cases we have patients who are diagnosed within a year. A total of 29% of the cases were diagnosed after a year. Out of these 92 cases of delayed diagnosis, we have 24 cases who have delayed the treatment also for more than a year. As shown in Figure 9, 1 refers to chemotherapy (CT), 2 refers to radiotherapy (RT), and 3 refers to surgery. Also it was seen that except for two cases all others

TABLE 4 Type of Cancer in Respondents

SN	Type of Cancer	Percentage
1	Blood	0.3
2	Bone	2.6
3	Brain	1.3
4	Breast	25
5	Colon	3.8
6	Ear	0.3
7	Endocrine	3.8
8	Gastrointestinal	9.6
9	Neck	1.6
10	Oral	25.6
11	Prostate	1.3
12	Respiratory	8.7
13	Skin	2.9
14	Spinal Cord	1.6
15	Testes	1
16	Urinary Bladder	1.6
17	Uterus	9

have to go for surgery along with CT or RT. Out of these 24 patients, 1 was very critical. Out of chronic patients, we have 11 patients who had a recurrence of cancer.

The recurrence phenomenon was highly observed in breast cancer patients followed by uterus, colon, skin, and oral cancer. The recurrence has a range of 2 years to 16 years.

5.2.6 Cancer Type and Gender

Though the data is small, it represents the findings which are supported by the literature. Among females, cases of breast cancer are prevalent, whereas in males the highest cases of oral cancer are found. In Figure 10, 1.0 represents male and 2.0 represents female.

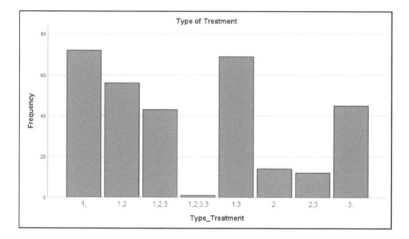

FIGURE 9   Frequency distribution of treatment type.

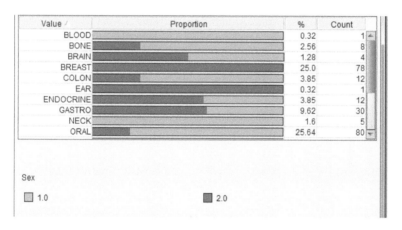

FIGURE 10   Distribution of cancer type and gender.

5.2.7 Cancer Type and Education (A Normalized Display)

Figure 11 depicts the normalized display of cancer type and education. Though the data is small we see that the detailed education distribution of only 50% are suffering from oral and breast cancer; then we see that the level of education is very poor. Illiteracy is high in both cases and the graduation level is low. This is because a majority of

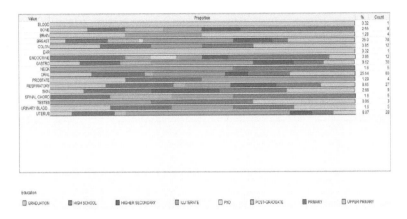

FIGURE 11 Education-wise distribution of cancer.

the population is coming from the rural background and a low-income strata.

5.3 Scenario-1 Analysis

This is the round one of data collection, and patients were asked how they felt at the initial stage when they were diagnosed with cancer and their present status with the treatment.

5.3.1 Physical Well-Being

The physical well-being (F1) construct is measured by nine items, which are fatigue (R1), appetite change (R2), pain (R3), sleep change (R4), weight change (R5), constipation (R6), nausea (R7), menstrual change (R8), and overall physical health (G9).

Thus we see from Table 5 that though overall health is not reported very bad by most respondents, other physical parameters are severely affected in about 60% of the respondents. Fatigue, change in appetite, suffering with pain, changes in sleep, weight loss, constipation, and nausea have affected severely (50–60%) to moderately (15–25%) all the patients.

TABLE 5   Status of Physical Well-Being

SN	Item (F1)	Mild %	Moderate %	Severe %
1	Fatigue (R1)	22.7	22.1	55.2
2	Appetite change (R2)	21.8	20.8	57.4
3	Pain (R3)	26.3	21.8	51.9
4	Sleep change (R4)	33.6	16.7	49.7
5	Weight change (R5)	18.6	25	56.4
6	Constipation (R6)	21.7	24.1	54.2
7	Nausea (R7)	24.4	16.3	59.3
8	Menstrual change (R8)	26.9	12.2	60.9
9	Overall physical health (G9)	30.4	39.7	29.9

5.3.2 Psychological Well-Being

The psychological well-being (F2) construct is measured by 17 items, which are difficulty in coping with disease (R10), difficulty in coping with treatment (R11), deterioration in life quality (R12), feeling of unhappiness (R13), lack of control (Psy14), no satisfaction from life (Psy15), loss of memory (Psy16), non-usefulness (Psy17), appearance change (R18), self-concept change (Psy19), initial diagnosis problem (R20), chemotherapy problem (R21), radiation problem (R22), surgery problem (R23), post-treatment problem (R24), anxiety (R25), and depression (R26) (Table 6).

Thus we see that many respondents were not able to cope with the disease (81.1%) at the initial stage and also with treatment (81.7%) in the beginning. Around 68% of the patients reported that there is a severe deterioration in their life quality. Fifty per cent of the patients were affected by the change in their appearance, especially weight loss at the initial stage. As the patients were diagnosed with cancer, they suffered severe anxiety (78.8%) and depression (78.5%). The reason cited by the majority of patients was that they will die very soon, as there is no cure for cancer, and even if they survive they will live a very miserable life.

TABLE 6 Status of Psychological Well-Being

SN	Item (F1)	Mild %	Moderate %	Severe %
1	Difficulty in coping with disease (R10)	18.9	15.3	81.1
2	Difficulty in coping with treatment (R11)	4.5	13.8	81.7
3	Deterioration in life quality (R12)	11.3	20.8	67.9
4	Feeling of unhappiness (R13)	11.3	17.9	70.8
5	Lack of control (Psy14)	28.4	32.5	39.1
6	No satisfaction from life (Psy15)	29.2	39.4	31.4
7	Loss of memory (Psy16)	22.5	30.4	47.1
8	Non-usefulness (Psy17)	38.1	45.9	16.0
9	Appearance change (R18)	24.6	25.7	49.7
10	Self-concept change (Psy19)	16.7	47.7	35.6
11	Initial diagnosis problem (R20)	8.3	27.3	64.4
12	Chemotherapy problem (R21)	27.5	18.3	54.2
13	Radiation problem (R22)	70.5	12.2	17.3
14	Surgery problem (R23)	53.3	8.2	38.5
15	Post-treatment problem (R24)	10	77.2	12.8
16	Anxiety (R25)	5.2	16.0	78.8
17	Depression (R26)	6.7	14.8	78.5

5.3.3 Fearfulness

The fearfulness (F3) construct is measured by five items, which are fear of future tests (R27), second cancer (R28), recurrence (R29), spreading (R30), and feeling normal (Fr31).

TABLE 7   Status of Fearfulness

SN	Item (F1)	Mild %	Moderate %	Severe %
1	Fear of future tests (R27)	1.3	13.8	84.9
2	Second cancer (R28)	2	10.5	87.5
3	Recurrence (R29)	1.9	9.0	89.1
4	Spreading (R30)	2.5	8.1	89.4
5	Feeling normal (Fr31)	30.7	38.5	30.8

From Table 7, we can see that fear is playing a very vital role in cancer patients. Nearly 90% of the patients are in fear of either recurrence of cancer or spreading of cancer. A reported 87.5% have fear of a second cancer. Also we see that 85% of the patients have a fear of future tests. Respondents are not very positive about feeling normal once cancer had occurred. Fear in the case of cancer patients is becoming a silent killer as observed during the survey.

5.3.4 Social Well-Being

The social well-being (F4) construct is measured by eight items, which are distress for family (Soc32), family support (Soc33), personal relationship (R34), sex life (R35), job (R36), household activities (R37), isolation (R38), and financial burden (R39).

From Table 8 it is evident that nearly 72.4% of the patients reported that cancer has very adversely hampered their household activities, whereas 67.9% reported that their job is very badly affected. Financial burden is increased to a large extent due to disease as reported by 69.2% of the cancer patients. Mostly the respondents have reported that sex life is affected, and 66% reported that cancer had a major impact on their sexual life. Nearly 56.4% feel severe isolation due to cancer. Personal relationships are adversely affected to a great extent, as reported by 54.8% of the cancer patients. A reported 36.9% of the patients reported that family support is not

TABLE 8   Status of Physical Well-Being

SN	Item (F1)	Mild %	Moderate %	Severe %
1	Distress for family (Soc32)	51.3	39.1	9.6
2	Family support (Soc33)	32.4	30.7	36.9
3	Personal relationship (R34)	19.2	26	54.8
4	Sex life (R35)	11.2	22.8	66
5	Job (R36)	13.1	19.0	67.9
6	Household activities (R37)	5.8	21.8	72.4
7	Isolation (R38)	15.4	28.2	56.4
8	Financial burden (R39)	6.7	24.1	69.2

adequate, whereas 32.4% reported it was more or less adequate. Nearly 51.3% of the respondents said that their family is not that much distressed with their disease, and only 9.6% said that the family is highly distressed.

5.3.5 Spiritual Well-Being

The spiritual well-being (F5) construct is measured by seven items, which are religious activities (Spr40), meditation (Spr41), spiritual change (Spr42), uncertainty (R43), positive change (Spr44), purpose of life (Spr45), and hope (Spr46).

We see from Table 9 that around 67% reported about the high uncertainty of their future. Only 38.1% reported that the disease has brought high positive change in their life, whereas 46.8% reported a moderate positive change in their life. Nearly 36.2% of patients said that prayer and meditation are highly important for them now, whereas 45.9% believe it is only moderately important to them. Nearly 46% of respondents said that the disease has brought moderate change in their spiritual life, whereas 31.7% agreed that it has brought a big change in their

TABLE 9   Status of Spiritual Well-Being

SN	Item (F1)	Mild %	Moderate %	Severe %
1	Religious activities (Spr40)	21.2	44.2	34.6
2	Meditation (Spr41)	19.9	43.9	36.2
3	Spiritual change (Spr42)	22.4	45.9	31.7
4	Uncertainty (R43)	10.6	22.4	67.0
5	Positive change (Spr44)	15.1	46.8	38.1
6	Purpose of life (Spr45)	32.1	49.6	18.3
7	Hope (Spr46)	25.3	45.5	29.2

spiritual life. After the occurrence of cancer respondents were asked whether they still feel their life purposeful; only 18.3% still feel very purposeful, only 49.6% felt moderately purposeful, and 32.1% feel not at all purposeful. A reported 29.2% are very hopeful even after suffering from cancer, but 45.5% of respondents are somewhat hopeful and 25.3% have lost their hope.

Hypothesis-1

H$_{01}$: QOL index has no correlation with age

After calculating the QoL index as shown in Table 10, we calculated the correlation coefficient between age and QoL index. The value of the correlation coefficient was 0.00039; thus, our null hypothesis is accepted showing no correlation between both the variables.

TABLE 10   QoL Index

	Category of QoL	Count	%
1	Less than 0.3	5	1.60
2	Less than 0.4	79	25.32
3	Less than 0.5	169	54.16
4	Less than 0.6	50	16.02
5	Greater than 0.6	9	2.89

Also the coefficient of association chi square (χ^2) was calculated to see if any association exists between two attributes. The calculated value of the test statistic was 3.802, and the tabulated value at 5% level of significance was 12.6. Thus, we accept the null hypothesis assuming that there is no association between age and QoL index.

5.4 Confirmatory Factor Analysis (CFA)

The next step was to conduct confirmatory factor analysis (CFA).

5.4.1 Physical Well-Being

The physical well-being (F1) construct is measured by nine items, and the factor analysis was done for the same.

Figure 12 shows the factor loading for each item and the fitness indexes for the physical well-being latent exogenous variable. All the items except R8 had factor loading more than 0.60, and hence only R8 will be deleted.

However, the fitness index shown previously suggests that the measurement model is insignificant due to some items having high correlated errors. So to achieve the fitness of the model, the Modification Index (MI) was examined

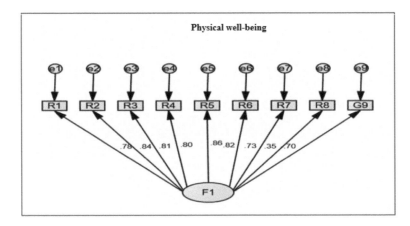

FIGURE 12 Network diagram (physical well-being).

TABLE 11   Summary of CFA for Physical Well-Being

Model Fit Summary	
Chi sq	382.736
DF	27
Chi sq/DF	14.175
GFI	0.789
AGFI	0.648
CFI	0.827
RMSE	0.206

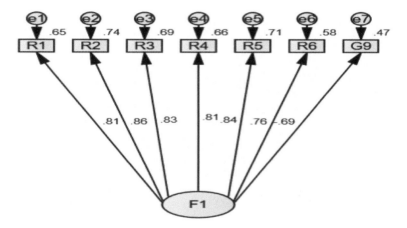

FIGURE 13   Network diagram for physical well-being (updated).

through Table 11. The items with high correlation (MI >15) in the measurement errors were eliminated or they were set as a free parameter estimate from the correlated pair. Thus, we eliminated R7, and the model fitness was achieved. The new fitness summary is given in Figure 13.

5.4.2 Psychological Well-Being

The psychological well-being (F2) construct is measured by 17 items, and the factor analysis was done for the same. Figure 14 shows the factor loading for each item for the psychological well-being latent exogenous variable. The

TABLE 12   Summary Table for CFA (Updated)

Model Fit Summary

Chi sq	73.489
DF	14
Chi sq/DF	5.249
GFI	0.934
AGFI	0.868
CFI	0.961
RMSE	0.117

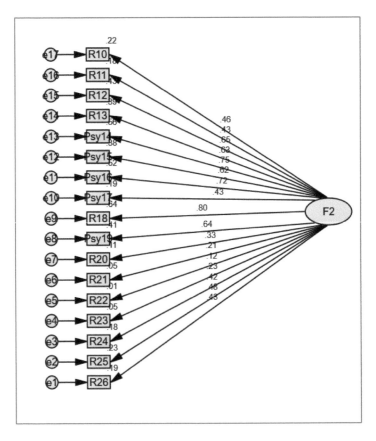

FIGURE 14   Network diagram for psychological factors.

TABLE 13 Model Summary (Psychological Factors)

Model Fit Summary	
Chi sq	1481.736
DF	119
Chi sq/DF	12.452
GFI	0.604
AGFI	0.490
CFI	0.469
RMSE	0.192

items having factor loading above 0.6 were selected for model fit. In all we have seven items that are extracted by the model, and they are R12, R13, Psy14, Psy15, Psy16, Psy17, R18, and Psy19. All the other 10 items having a factor loading less than 0.60 are deleted from the model.

However, the fitness index in Table 12 suggested that the measurement model is insignificant due to some items having high correlated errors. So to achieve the fitness of the model the MI was examined. The items with high correlation (MI >15) in the measurement errors were eliminated or they were set as a free parameter estimate from the correlated pair. Thus, we eliminated Psy14, Psy15, Psy16, and Psy17 from the model shown in Tables 13 and 14 to achieve fitness. The new fitness summary is given in Figure 15.

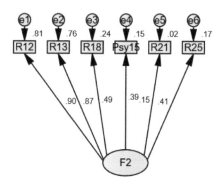

FIGURE 15 Updated network diagram (psychological factors).

TABLE 14   Model Fit Psychological (Updated)

Model Fit Summary	
Chi sq	100.189
DF	9
Chi sq/DF	11.132
GFI	0.917
AGFI	0.806
CFI	0.837
RMSE	0.180

5.4.3 Fearfulness

The fearfulness (F3) construct is measured by five items, and the factor analysis was done for the same. Figure 16 shows the factor loading for each item for the fearfulness latent exogenous variable.

All the items except Fr31 had factor loading more than 0.60, and hence only Fr31 will be deleted. The model fit summary is given in Table 15.

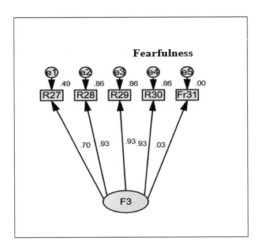

FIGURE 16   Network diagram for fearfulness.

TABLE 15   Model Summary (Fearfulness)

Model Fit Summary

Chi sq	51.261
DF	5
Chi sq/DF	10.312
GFI	0.937
AGFI	0.811
CFI	0.959
RMSE	0.173

5.4.4 Social Well-Being

The social well-being (F4) construct is measured by eight items, and the factor analysis was done for the same. Figure 17 shows the factor loading for each item for the social well-being latent exogenous variable. We have only four items, viz; R36, R37, R38, and R39 with negative feeling, as seen in the figure. All four items have factor loading less than 0.60 and were deleted from the model. The model summary is given in Table 16.

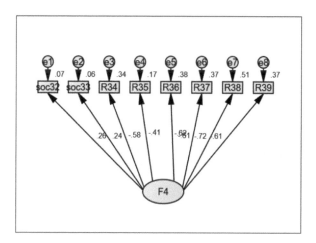

FIGURE 17   Network diagram for social well-being.

TABLE 16 Model Summary (Social Well-Being)

Model Fit Summary	
Chi sq	281.433
DF	20
Chi sq/DF	14.072
GFI	0.815
AGFI	0.667
CFI	0.604
RMSE	0.205

However, the fitness index in the model suggests that the measurement model is insignificant due to some items having high correlated errors. So to achieve the fitness of the model the MI was examined. The items with high correlation (MI >15) in the measurement errors were eliminated or they were set as a free parameter estimate from the correlated pair. Thus, we eliminated R34, Soc32, and Soc33 from the model to achieve fitness. The new fitness summary is given in Table 17 and Figure 18.

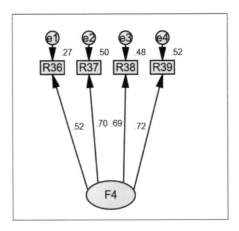

FIGURE 18 Network diagram for social well-being (updated).

TABLE 17   Model Summary for Social Well-Being (Updated)

Model Fit Summary	
Chi sq	4.414
DF	2
Chi sq/DF	2.207
GFI	0.993
AGFI	0.965
CFI	0.991
RMSE	0.062

5.4.5 Spiritual Well-Being

The spiritual well-being (F5) construct is measured by seven items, and the factor analysis was done for the same. Figure 20 shows the factor loading for each item for the spiritual well-being latent exogenous variable. We have only three items, viz; Spr40, Spr41, Spr42 and Spr44 selected by the model, as seen in the Figure 19. All four items have factor loading less than 0.60 and were deleted from the model. The model summary is given in Table 18.

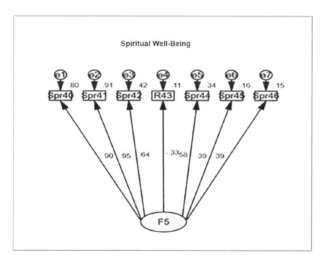

FIGURE 19   Network diagram for spiritual well-being.

TABLE 18 Model Summary (Spiritual Well-Being)

Model Fit Summary	
Chi sq	280.42
DF	14
Chi sq/DF	20.030
GFI	0.798
AGFI	0.595
CFI	0.749
RMSE	0.247

However, the fitness index in the table and the model suggest that the measurement model is insignificant due to some items having high correlated errors. So to achieve the fitness of the model the MI was examined. The items with high correlation (MI >15) in the measurement errors were eliminated or they were set as a free parameter estimate from the correlated pair. Thus, we eliminated R43, Spr45, and Spr46 from the model to achieve fitness. The new fitness summary is given in Table 19.

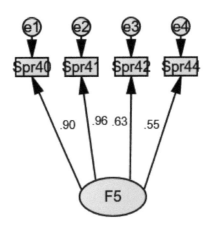

FIGURE 20 Network diagram for spiritual well-being (updated).

TABLE 19 Updated Model Summary (Spiritual Well-Being)

Model Fit Summary

Chi sq	19.998
DF	2
Chi sq/DF	9.999
GFI	0.972
AGFI	0.861
CFI	0.974
RMSE	0.170

5.5 The Measurement Model for QoL

After the selection of relevant exogenous variables through CFA, the next step was to proceed with SEM. The results of the same are displayed in Figure 21. The model summary is also displayed in Table 20.

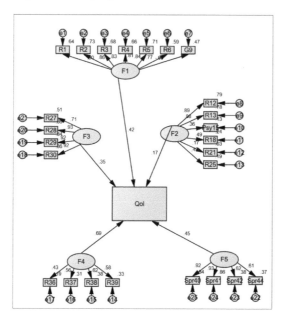

FIGURE 21 QoL model.

TABLE 20   Model Fit Summary (QoL)

Model Fit Summary	
Chi sq	1635.916
DF	296
Chi sq/DF	5.527
GFI	0.705
AGFI	0.650
CFI	0.763
RMSE	0.121

Now the redundant items in the initial fit model were examined through the MI table which is produced by SEM. The most highly correlated pair of items that are greater than 15 will be set as a free parameter estimate or

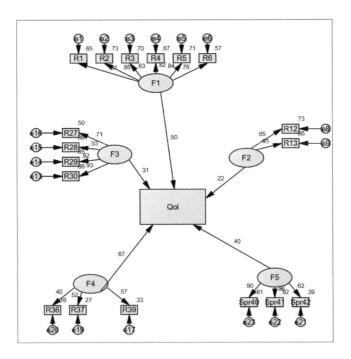

FIGURE 22   QoL network diagram (updated).

TABLE 21 MODEL FIT SUMMARY (UPDATED MODEL)

Model Fit Summary

Chi sq	432.346
DF	13
Chi sq/DF	3.3
GFI	0.905
AGFI	0.860
CFI	0.924
RMSE	0.086

one item will be deleted. The model is specified until uni-dimensionality for the model is achieved through a fitness check. The variables Psy15 and R25 were deleted from construct F2. R37 and R38 were deleted from construct F4. Spr44 was deleted from construct F5. After deleting these exogenous variables, the fitness indexes for the model were achieved as shown in Figure 23. The model summary is also displayed in Table 21.

5.6 Structural Equation Model

The standardised regression weights explained the relationship of each of the items with the variable; when F1 goes up by 1 standard deviation, QoL goes up by 0.569 standard deviation, and when F2 goes up by 1 standard deviation, QoL goes up by 0.222 standard deviation. When F3 goes up by 1 standard deviation, QoL goes up by 0.354 standard deviation. When F4 goes up by 1 standard deviation, QoL goes up by 0.431 standard deviation. When F5 goes up by 1 standard deviation, QoL goes up by 0.322 standard deviation. Further, the correlation between the latent construct F1 and QoL is estimated to be 0.569, between latent construct F2 and QoL is estimated to be 0.222, between latent construct F3 and QoL is estimated to be 0.354, between latent construct F4 and QoL is estimated to be 0.431, and finally between latent construct F5 and QoL is estimated to be 0.322. Analysis shows that items R1, R2, R3, R4, R5, and R6 significantly contribute to F1; items R12 and R13 significantly contribute to F2; and items R27, R28, R29, and R30 significantly contribute to F3, but items R36 and R39 are not contributing significantly to F4 in the final model, though in individual CFA for each exogenous variable, they were significantly contributing. We have included it in the model as the model fit indexes are achieved. Items Spr40, Spr41, and Spr42 significantly contribute to F5. Analysis for individual regression weights showed that each item is highly significant where the p-value is less than 0.0001. It was estimated that QoL explains 57.0% of its variance, which means that the error variance of QoL is approximately 43.0% of the variance itself. All relationships were found to be significant since the p-values are less than 0.001. Moreover, the hypothesis for variance concluded that the variance for all variables in the model is significantly different from zero. Hence, we can conclude the model fit was statistically significant. Finally, the overall fitness is assessed using absolute fit, incremental fit, and parsimonious fit. According to Figure 22 and Table 21, the values of model performance indicators such as RMSEA = 0.088, CFI = 0.924, TLI = 0.911, GFI = 0.905, and Chi sq/DF = 3.3 indicate that all indicators are significant and achieved the model criteria. The measurement equation models identified are:

Physical well-being (exogenous) variable:

$$R1 = 0.76 * F1 + 0.65$$

$$R2 = 0.84 * F1 + 0.73$$

$$R3 = 0.82 * F1 + 0.70$$

$$R4 = 0.84 * F1 + 0.67$$

$$R5 = 0.85 * F1 + 0.71$$
$$R6 = 0.81 * F1 + 0.57$$

Psychological well-being (exogenous) variable:

$$R12 = 0.82 * F2 + 0.73$$
$$R13 = 0.84 * F2 + 0.86$$

Fear (exogenous) variable:

$$R27 = 0.71 * F3 + 0.50$$
$$R28 = 0.93 * F3 + 0.86$$
$$R29 = 0.92 * F3 + 0.85$$
$$R30 = 0.93 * F3 + 0.86$$

Social well-being (exogenous) variable:

$$R36 = 0.40 * F4 + 0.16$$
$$R37 = 0.52 * F4 + 0.27$$
$$R39 = 0.57 * F4 + 0.33$$

Spiritual well-being (exogenous) variable:

$$Spr40 = 0.89 * F5 + 0.81$$
$$Spr41 = 0.97 * F5 + 0.92$$
$$Spr42 = 0.63 * F5 + 0.39$$

The structural equation model can be written as:

$$QoL = 0.50 * F1 + 0.22 * F2 + 0.31 * F3 + 0.67 * F4 + 0.40 * F5$$

1. H_{02}: Factors affecting QoL are associated with patient well-being

Hence, from SEM we can say all factors are playing their role in affecting QoL. Thus, it can be seen that fearfulness plays a very pivotal role in the assessment of

QoL of cancer patients. As soon as the patient is diagnosed with cancer, he or she feels that life is coming to an end and nothing can save them. They start suffering from high anxiety, depression, and sleeplessness. Fear psychosis develops in these patients very fast, and they need counselling from family, friends, and above all from a professional counsellor. The second important factor directly impacting QoL is physical well-being because pain, loss of appetite, nausea, fatigue, and other physical deterioration parameters directly affect physical health. Social well-being is also affected, as personal relationships and family stress also affect QoL.

5.7 Scenario-2 Analysis

This is round two of data collection, and patients were asked how they felt after 6 months of follow-up treatment. Due to a lack of time and money, more follow-ups could not be done.

5.7.1 Physical Well-Being

After undergoing 6 months of treatment, we see that the severity of various indicators like fatigue, appetite change, pain, nausea, constipation, etc., has reduced to some extent, as shown in Table 22. Most respondents reported that treatment has been able to reduce their misery to a large extent (40%) and in some to a moderate level (35%). Thus we see that nearly 25% of the respondents have a mild effect, and the reason was that they were suffering from grade III or grade IV cancer.

5.7.2 Psychological Well-Being

There was a visible change in psychological parameters after 6 months follow-up treatment (Table 23). Though there is no formal counselling cell for the cancer patients, doctors at their individual level try to counsel patients on various problems faced by them. Thus, we see the percentage drop in the patient category of 'not able to cope with

TABLE 22 Status of Physical Well-Being

SN	Item (F1)	Mild %	Moderate %	Severe %
1	Fatigue (R1)	29.7	34.96	35.34
2	Appetite change (R2)	27.44	31.23	41.35
3	Pain (R3)	28.9	26.4	44.7
4	Sleep change (R4)	19.5	28.6	51.87
5	Weight change (R5)	19.5	31.58	40.23
6	Constipation (R6)	31.58	24.06	44.36
7	Nausea (R7)	31.58	28.20	40.23
8	Menstrual change (R8)	15.79	18.05	66.16
9	Overall physical health (G9)	54.5	27.07	18.42

the disease' reduced drastically (from 81.1% to 7.9%). The same scenario was apparent for 'difficulty in coping with treatment' (from 81.7% to 11.65%). The main reason was counselling by doctors and family members. The symptoms of severe anxiety and depression reduced from 78.8% and 78.5% to 13.53% and 16.54%, respectively. Feelings of unhappiness reduced drastically from 70.8% to 21.81%.

TABLE 23 Status of Psychological Well-Being

SN	Item (F1)	Mild %	Moderate %	Severe %
1	Difficulty in coping with disease (R10)	54.89	36.85	7.90
2	Difficulty in coping with treatment (R11)	54.5	33.84	11.65
3	Deterioration in life quality (R12)	39.48	39.10	21.42
4	Feeling of unhappiness (R13)	39.48	38.72	21.81

(Continued)

TABLE 23 (Continued)

SN	Item (F1)	Mild %	Moderate %	Severe %
5	Lack of control (Psy14)	66.92	25.57	7.51
6	No satisfaction from life (Psy15)	53.00	33.08	13.91
7	Loss of memory (Psy16)	68.79	22.94	8.27
8	Non-usefulness (Psy17)	37.97	35.72	26.32
9	Appearance change (R18)	32.70	45.48	21.80
10	Self-concept change (Psy19)	51.13	38.35	10.53
11	Initial diagnosis problem (R20)	37.59	35.71	15.04
12	Chemotherapy problem (R21)	48.50	25.56	25.94
13	Radiation problem (R22)	15.04	20.68	64.29
14	Surgery problem (R23)	31.58	19.17	49.25
15	Post-treatment problem (R24)	45.86	38.72	15.41
16	Anxiety (R25)	53.38	33.08	13.53
17	Depression (R26)	50.00	33.46	16.54

5.7.3 Fearfulness

The fearfulness (F3) construct is measured by five items, which are fear of future tests (R27), second cancer (R28), recurrence (R29), spreading (R30), and feeling normal (Fr31).

Thus we see from Table 24 that fear is playing a very vital role in cancer patients' lives. Nearly 90% of the

TABLE 24   Status of Fearfulness

SN	Item (F1)	Mild %	Moderate %	Severe %
1	Fear of future tests (R27)	62.78	28.20	9.02
2	Second cancer (R28)	65.41	24.44	10.15
3	Recurrence (R29)	66.17	24.82	9.02
4	Spreading (R30)	66.54	24.07	9.40
5	Feeling normal (Fr31)	51.51	27.44	21.05

patients were in fear of either recurrence of cancer or spreading of cancer; now this percentage reduced to 9% only. The fear of a second cancer reduced from 87.5% to 10.15% cases only. Fear of future tests reduced from 85% to 9.02%.

5.7.4 Social Well-Being

The social well-being (F4) construct (Table 25) is measured by eight items, which are distress for the family (Soc32), family support (Soc33), personal relationships (R34), sex life (R35), job (R36), household activities (R37), isolation (R38), and financial burden (R39).

Nearly 72.4% of the patients reported that cancer has very adversely hampered their household activities, but after

TABLE 25   Status of Social Well-Being

SN	Item (F1)	Mild %	Moderate %	Severe %
1	Distress for the family (Soc32)	56.3	38.2	5.5
2	Family support (Soc33)	48.88	30.82	20.30
3	Personal relationships (R34)	33.08	39.10	27.18
4	Sex life (R35)	39.10	34.97	25.94
5	Job (R36)	36.10	29.70	34.22
6	Household activities (R37)	49.24	33.84	16.92
7	Isolation (R38)	28.95	40.23	30.83
8	Financial burden (R39)	16.17	35.34	48.50

treatment and follow-up this reduced to 16.92% only. The effect on a person's job reduced from 67.9% to 34.22% after follow-up and treatment. The financial burden remained more or less the same, as cancer treatment is costly. The effect on sex life reduced from 66% to 25.94%. In both scenarios, family distress remains the same as shown in table 25. The feeling of isolation reduced from 56.4% to 30.83%.

5.7.5 Spiritual Well-Being

The spiritual well-being (F5) construct is measured by seven items, which are religious activities (Spr40), meditation (Spr41), spiritual change (Spr42), uncertainty (R43), positive change (Spr44), purpose of life (Spr45), and hope (Spr46).

Thus we see from Table 26 that around 28.20% reported on the high uncertainty of their future, which was around 67% at the initial stage of cancer detection. Nearly 36.2% of patients said that prayer and meditation are highly important for them now, and this increased to 45.14%. Religious activities also increased mildly. Hopefulness in life increased from 29.2% to 53.76%.

The QoL Index as seen in Table 27 also changed after treatment and some basic counselling given by doctors, family, and friends. As there was no formal counselling,

TABLE 26   Status of Spiritual Well-Being

SN	Item (F1)	Mild %	Moderate %	Severe %
1	Religious activities (Spr40)	30.02	34.22	35.76
2	Meditation (Spr41)	20.27	34.59	45.14
3	Spiritual change (Spr42)	50.00	30.08	19.93
4	Uncertainty (R43)	42.86	28.95	28.20
5	Positive change (Spr44)	59.03	30.83	10.16
6	Purpose of life (Spr45)	41.36	29.70	28.95
7	Hope (Spr46)	18.8	27.45	53.76

TABLE 27 QoL Index

	Category of QoL	Count	%
1	Less than 0.3	7	2.6
2	Less than 0.4	24	9.02
3	Less than 0.5	78	29.32
4	Less than 0.6	117	43.98
5	Less than 0.7	37	13.91
6	Greater than 0.7	3	1.13

the change was very low, but the encouraging picture is that it was in a positive direction.

5.8 Confirmatory Factor Analysis (CFA)

The next step was to conduct CFA.

5.8.1 Physical Well-Being

The physical well-being (F1) construct is measured by nine items, and the CFA was done for the same. Figure 23 shows the factor loading for each item. All the items except R8 had factor loading more than 0.60, and hence only R8 will be deleted. Also G9 has negative factor loading.

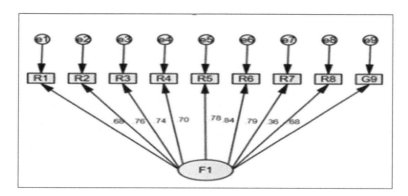

FIGURE 23 CFA (physical well-being).

TABLE 28   CFA Fit Summary (Physical Well-Being)

Model Fit Summary

Chi sq	308.789
DF	27
Chi sq/DF	11.437
GFI	0.775
AGFI	0.625
CFI	0.803
RMSE	0.198

The fitness index of the model in Table 28 suggests that the measurement model is insignificant due to some items having high correlated errors. So to achieve the fitness of the model the MI was examined. The items with high correlation (MI >15) in the measurement errors were eliminated or they were set as a free parameter estimate from the correlated pair. Thus, we eliminated R6 and R8 and the model fitness was achieved. The new fitness summary is given in Table 29 and Figure 24.

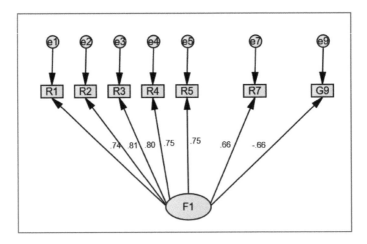

FIGURE 24   CFA physical well-being (updated).

TABLE 29   CFA Fit for Physical Well-Being (Updated)

Model Fit Summary	
Chi sq	87.574
DF	14
Chi sq/DF	6.255
GFI	0.903
AGFI	0.807
CFI	0.924
RMSE	0.141

5.8.2 Psychological Well-Being

The psychological well-being (F2) construct is measured by 17 items, and the factor analysis was done for the same. Figure 25 shows the factor loading for each item for the

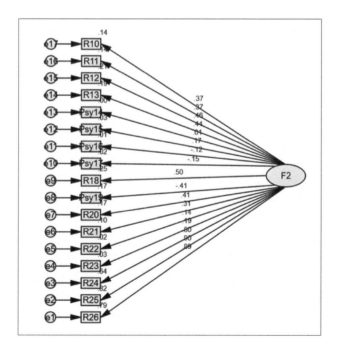

FIGURE 25   CFA diagram psychological well-being.

psychological well-being latent exogenous variable. The item having factor loading above 0.60 has both a positive feeling and negative feeling. To get better effective results, both are analysed. In all we have eight items that are extracted by the model. We have three items, viz; R12, R13, and R18 with a positive feeling as seen in Figure 25, whereas we have five items, viz; Psy14, Psy15, Psy16, Psy17, Psy19, that have a negative feeling. All nine items having factor loading less than 0.60 and will be deleted from the model.

The fitness index of the model in Table 30 suggests that the measurement model is insignificant due to some items having

TABLE 30 CFA Fit Summary (Psychological Well-Being)

Model Fit Summary	
Chi sq	308.789
DF	27
Chi sq/DF	11.437
GFI	0.775
AGFI	0.625
CFI	0.803
RMSE	0.198

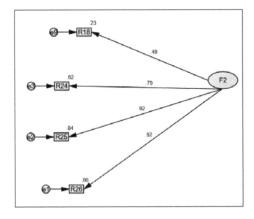

FIGURE 26   CFA diagram psychological well-being (updated).

TABLE 31   CFA Fit Psychological Well-Being (Updated)

Model Fit Summary

Chi sq	7.764
DF	2
Chi sq/DF	3.882
GFI	0.986
AGFI	0.929
CFI	0.991
RMSE	0.104

high correlated errors. So to achieve fitness of the model the MI was examined. The items with high correlation (MI >15) in the measurement errors were eliminated or they were set as a free parameter estimate from the correlated pair. But to achieve model fitness, we have to introduce R18 with loading less than 0.6 but highest in the eliminated group. The new fitness summary is given in Table 31 and Figure 26.

5.8.3 Fearfulness

The fearfulness (F3) construct is measured by five items, and the factor analysis was done for the same. Figure 27 shows the factor loading for each item for the fearfulness latent

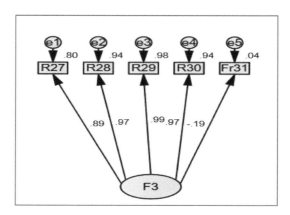

FIGURE 27   CFA diagram fearfulness.

TABLE 32 CFA Summary (Fearfulness)

Model Fit Summary	
Chi sq	59.802
DF	5
Chi sq/DF	11.960
GFI	0.932
AGFI	0.796
CFI	0.969
RMSE	0.203

exogenous variable. All the items except Fr31 had factor loading more than 0.60, and hence only Fr31 will be deleted. The model fitness index as seen in Table 32 is achieved.

5.8.4 Social Well-Being

The social well-being (F4) construct is measured by eight items, and the factor analysis was done for the same. Figure 28 shows the factor loading for each item for the social well-being latent exogenous variable. We have only

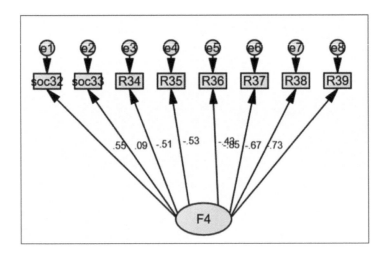

FIGURE 28 CFA diagram (social well-being).

TABLE 33 CFA Summary (Social Well-Being)

Model Fit Summary

Chi sq	281.433
DF	20
Chi sq/DF	14.072
GFI	0.815
AGFI	0.667
CFI	0.604
RMSE	0.205

three items, viz; R37, R38, and R39 with a negative feel-ing as seen in Figure 28. The remaining five items having factor loading less than 0.60 and were deleted from the model. The model summary is given in Table 33.

However, the fitness index in the model suggests that the measurement model is insignificant due to some items having high correlated errors. So to achieve the fitness of the model the MI was examined. The items with high correlation (MI >15) in the measurement errors were eliminated or they were set as a free parameter estimate from the correlated pair. So to achieve the fitness index

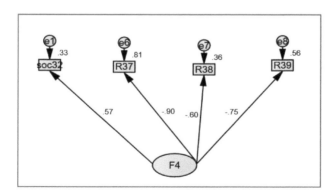

FIGURE 29 CFA diagram social well-being (updated).

TABLE 34   CFA Summary Social Well-Being (Updated)

Model Fit Summary	
Chi sq	35.458
DF	2
Chi sq/DF	17.729
GFI	0.944
AGFI	0.719
CFI	0.911
RMSE	0.251

we introduced Soc32 in the model. The new fitness summary is given in Table 34 and Figure 29.

5.8.5 Spiritual Well-Being

The spiritual well-being (F5) construct is measured by seven items, and the factor analysis was done for the same. Figure 30 shows the factor loading for each item for the spiritual well-being latent exogenous variable.

We have four items, viz; Spr40, Spr41, Spr42, and Spr45 selected by the model, as seen in Figure 30. The three items with factor loading less than 0.60 were deleted from the model. The model summary is given in Table 35.

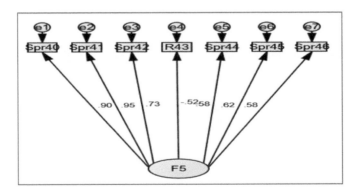

FIGURE 30   CFA diagram (spiritual well-being).

TABLE 35   CFA Summary (Spiritual Well-Being)

Model Fit Summary

Chi sq	437.203
DF	14
Chi sq/DF	31.229
GFI	0.684
AGFI	0.369
CFI	0.685
RMSE	0.338

However, the fitness index in the model suggests that the measurement model is insignificant due to some items having high correlated errors. So to achieve fitness of the model the MI was examined. The items with high correlation (MI >15) in the measurement errors were eliminated or they were set as a free parameter estimate from the correlated pair. Thus, we eliminated R43, Spr44, and Spr46 from the model to achieve fitness. The new fitness summary is given in Table 36 and Figure 31.

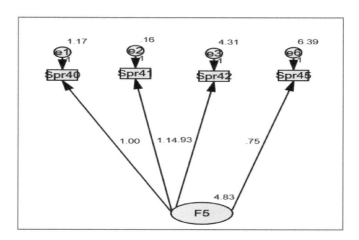

FIGURE 31   CFA diagram (updated) spiritual well-being.

TABLE 36   CFA Summary (Updated) Spiritual Well-Being

Model Fit Summary	
Chi sq	29.834
DF	2
Chi sq/DF	14.917
GFI	0.949
AGFI	0.744
CFI	0.960
RMSE	0.22

5.8.6 The Measurement Model for QoL

After selecting the relevant exogenous variables through CFA, the next step was to proceed with SEM. The results of the same are shown in Figures 32 and 33. The model summary is also displayed in Table 37 and Figure 32.

Now the redundant items in the initial fit model were examined through the MI table, which is produced by SEM. The most highly correlated pair of items which are greater than 15 will be set as a free parameter estimate or one item will be deleted. The model is specified until unidimensionality is achieved through fitness checking. The variables Psy15 and R25 were deleted from construct

TABLE 37   CFA Model Summary of QoL

Model Fit Summary	
Chi sq	1374.185
DF	249
Chi sq/DF	5.519
GFI	0.674
AGFI	0.608
CFI	0.808
RMSE	0.131

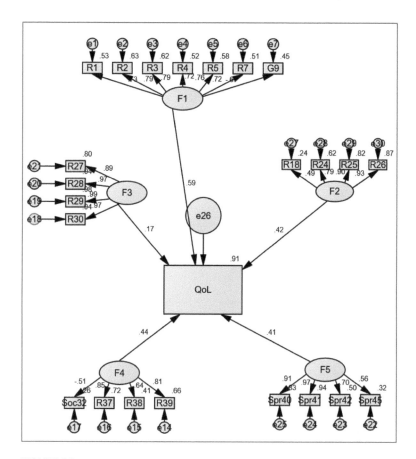

FIGURE 32 CFA model for QoL.

F2. R37 and R38 were deleted from construct F4. Spr44 was deleted from construct F5. After deleting these exogenous variables, the fitness indexes for the model were achieved as shown in Figure 33. The model summary is also displayed (see Table 36).

5.8.7 Structural Equation Model

The standardised regression weights explained the relationship of each item with the variable; when F1 goes up by 1 standard deviation, QoL goes up by 0.58 standard deviation, and when F2 goes up by 1 standard deviation,

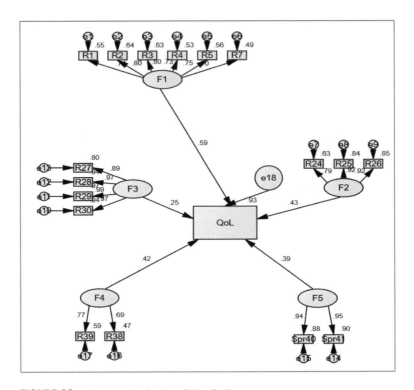

FIGURE 33 CFA model (updated) for QoL.

QoL goes up by 0.43 standard deviation. When F3 goes up by 1 standard deviation, QoL goes up by 0.25 standard deviation. When F4 goes up by 1 standard deviation, QoL goes up by 0.42 standard deviation. When F5 goes up by 1 standard deviation, QoL goes up by 0.39 standard deviation. Further, the correlation between latent construct F1 and QoL is estimated to be 0.589, between latent construct F2 and QoL is estimated to be 0.43, between latent construct F3 and QoL is estimated to be 0.25, between latent construct F4 and QoL is estimated to be 0.42, and finally between latent construct F5 and QoL is estimated to be 0.39. Analysis shows that items R1, R2, R3, R4, R5, and R7 significantly contribute to F1; items

R24, R25, and R26 significantly contribute to F2; and items R27, R28, R29, and R30 significantly contribute to F3, but item R38 is not contributing significantly to F4. However, R39 does significantly contribute to F4 in the final model, though in individual CFAs for each exogenous variable. Spr40 and Spr41 contribute significantly to F5. We have included it in the model, as the model fit indexes are achieved. Analysis for individual regression weights showed that each item is highly significant when the p-value is less than 0.0001. It was estimated that QoL explains 93.0% of its variance, which means that the error variance of QoL is approximately 0.07% of the variance itself. All relationships were found to be significant since the p-values are less than 0.001. Moreover, the hypothesis for variance concluded that the variance for all variables in the model is significantly different from zero. Hence, we can conclude the model fit was statistically significant.

Finally, the overall fitness is assessed using absolute fit, incremental fit, and parsimonious fit. According to Figure 33, the values of the model performance indicator such as RMSEA = 0.086, CFI = 0.924, TLI = 0.911, GFI= 0.905, and Chi-sq/DF = 3.3 indicate that all indicators are significant and achieved the model criteria as seen in Table 38.

TABLE 38   CFA Model Summary (Updated)

Model Fit Summary

Chi sq	432.346
DF	13
Chi sq/DF	3.3
GFI	0.905
AGFI	0.860
CFI	0.924
RMSE	0.086

The measurement equation models identified are:

Physical well-being (exogenous) variable:

$$R1 = 0.71 * F1 + 0.55$$
$$R2 = 0.80 * F1 + 0.64$$
$$R3 = 0.80 * F1 + 0.63$$
$$R4 = 0.73 * F1 + 0.53$$
$$R5 = 0.75 * F1 + 0.56$$
$$R7 = 0.70 * F1 + 0.49$$

Psychological well-being (exogenous) variable:

$$R24 = 0.79 * F2 + 0.63$$
$$R25 = 0.92 * F2 + 0.84$$
$$R25 = 0.92 * F2 + 0.85$$

Fear (exogenous) variable:

$$R27 = 0.80 * F3 + 0.89$$
$$R28 = 0.94 * F3 + 0.97$$
$$R29 = 0.97 * F3 + 0.99$$
$$R30 = 0.94 * F3 + 0.97$$

Social well-being (exogenous) variable:

$$R38 = 0.47 * F4 + 0.69$$
$$R39 = 0.59 * F4 + 0.77$$

Spiritual well-being (exogenous) variable:

$$Spr40 = 0.88 * F5 + 0.94$$
$$Spr41 = 0.90 * F5 + 0.95$$

The structural equation model can be written as:

$$QoL = 0.59 * F10.43 * F2 + 0.25 * F3 + 0.42 * F4 + 0.39 * F5$$

Thus it can be seen that the psychological factor along with fear constitute around 68%, and this is very high. After treatment and follow-up, we see that there is an increase in the psychological factor (43%) and social factor (42%) but the fear factor reduced slightly from 31% to 25%. Thus we see that after counselling and treatment, the prominent fear factor is reduced to a great extent. Before and after follow-up, no change was found in physical well-being because the physical symptoms remain more or less the same at the early stage of cancer and decline in the later stages.

CHAPTER 6

Result and Discussion

6.1 General Findings

- Around 67% of the population coming to a tertiary care hospital belongs to rural India. In Uttar Pradesh (UP), we have only three hospitals located in Lucknow with super-speciality services in cancer care. Some primary level of cancer treatment is done at Banaras Hindu University (BHU) hospital, but mainly patients are referred to the three hospitals. Also it is seen that people in the higher middle income class or upper income class, once diagnosed with cancer, prefer to go to Apollo Hospital, Delhi, or Tata Memorial Centre, Mumbai, one of the oldest cancer hospitals in India.

- The respondents coming to these hospitals are mostly (71.8%) from a lower income group. As they belong to a lower income group, they are more vulnerable to this disease. Most of the time due to a lack of funding, they cannot afford early treatment or the right treatment place.

- Money turns out to be an important factor in the delay of treatment.

- Out of 310 respondents we have 26.9% of the respondents who were illiterate. Only 23.7% of the respondents were either graduate level or above.

 DOI: 10.1201/9781003437994-6

Thus another important factor for delayed treatment turns out to be lower literacy levels, which give rise to lower awareness levels.

- The lower awareness level becomes a hurdle in achieving better quality of life.
- Female representation was 53%, while for men it was 47%. It could be inferred that we have a high prevalence of breast cancer in India due to which we had more female respondents.
- Mostly the respondents were married (89%).
- The female respondents made up 54%; hence, housewives constitute 39.1% of the occupational status basket. Another 28.8% are either self-employed or government employed or professionals; 9.3% are farmers and 17.3% of the respondents are either unemployed or labourers.
- Though the age distribution range is quite large i.e., 12–81 years, 53% of the respondents lie between the ages of 36 and 55 years. Thus we can also conclude that the middle-age group is more prone to cancer then elderly or very young patients. Also it is seen that if cancer occurs during this age group, than longevity is not ensured, or we may infer that the life expectancy is reduced due to cancer.
- The body mass index (BMI) status of 31.7% of the respondents was normal, whereas 16.7% of the population suffers from either type I, II, or III degree of malnourishment. A reported 26.9% were overweight, and only 7.4% were over obese. The major reason for a low BMI is that there is a sudden loss of weight due to the occurrence of cancer, on one hand, and also due to chemotherapy, on the other hand.
- The sample is truly representing the population status, as we have 25.6% of the patients suffering from oral cancer (the highest type of cancer often found in Indian males) and 25% of the patients suffering from breast cancer (mainly women). This is also supported by the finding of the National Institute

of Cancer Prevention and Research (NICPR) in that the maximum number of cases are reported to be suffering from oral and breast cancer in India. High preventive measures are needed in this area. Other types of cancers through which patients are majorly affected are gastrointestinal 9.6%, uterine 9%, and respiratory 9.6%. Patients suffering from blood, prostate, and ear cancers are very negligible: nearly 0.3%. Endocrine, colon, bone, and skin cancer also affect around 3–4% of the respondent population.

- It was good to know that in most of the cases we have patients who are diagnosed within a year. Twenty-nine per cent of the cases were diagnosed after a year. Out of these 92 cases of delayed diagnosis, we have 24 cases who have delayed treatment for more than a year.
- Aside from two cases, all other patients underwent surgery along with chemotherapy (CT) or radiation therapy (RT).
- Out of chronic patients we have 11 patients who have a recurrence of cancer. The recurrence phenomenon was highly observed in breast cancer patients followed by uterine, colon, skin, and oral cancer. The recurrence has the range of 2–16 years.

6.2 Scenario-1 Findings

- Nine items used to test physical well-being show that more than 50% of the respondents suffer severely with symptoms like fatigue, appetite change, pain, sleep and weight change, constipation, nausea, menstrual change, etc.
- Psychological well-being was measured by 17 items, and most of the respondents reported severe behaviour at onset. Around 81% of the respondents reported severe difficulty in coping with the disease or treatment at the initial stage.

- Around 78% of respondents reported severe anxiety and depression when they were diagnosed with cancer.
- Around 68% of the patients reported that there is severe deterioration in their quality of life, as now they feel unhappy and have a feeling of non-usefulness. The reason cited by the majority of patients was that they will have to lead a very miserable life.
- Due to weight loss at the initial stage, 55% of the patients were affected by the change in their appearance.
- More than 54% of the patients reported severe problem with chemotherapy, followed by surgery 38%. A reported 70.5% of the respondents reported mild problems with radiation treatment.
- Fear was measured by five items, and it turned out to be the biggest factor affecting quality of life in the whole study. The highest fear factor was of recurrence (89.1%) and spreading (89.4%). A reported 87.5% feared a second cancer, while 84.9% featured future test results.
- Social well-being was measured by eight items. Nearly 72.4% of the patients reported that cancer had adversely hampered their daily household activities, whereas 67.9% reported that their job is very badly affected leading to family tensions.
- An increase in financial burden to a large extent due to disease was reported by nearly 69.2% of the cancer patients.
- Mostly all reported that sex life was affected in one way or another, but out of these 66% reported that cancer had a major impact on their sexual life.
- Nearly 56.4% feel severe isolation due to cancer.
- Personal relationships were adversely affected, as reported by 54.8% of the cancer patients.
- A reported 36.9% of the patients said that family support is not adequate, whereas 32.4% reported family support was more or less adequate.

- Nearly 51.3% of the respondents said that their family was not very distressed with their disease, and only 9.6% said that their family was highly distressed.
- The spiritual well-being was measured using seven items. Around 67% of respondents reported the high uncertainty of their future life.
- Only 38.1% reported that the disease has brought a high positive change in their life, whereas 46.8% reported a moderate positive change in their life.
- Nearly 36.2% of patients said that prayer and meditation were highly important for them now, whereas 45.9% believed it was only moderately important to them.
- Nearly 46% of respondents said that the disease brought moderate change in their spiritual life, whereas 31.7% said it has brought a big change in their spiritual life.
- After the occurrence of cancer, respondents were asked whether they still feel life is purposeful; only 18.3% felt very purposeful still, but on the other hand only 49.6% moderately felt the same, and 32.1% felt that life was no longer purposeful.
- Only 29.2% reported high hope even after suffering from cancer, but 45.5% of respondents were somewhat hopeful and 25.3% were not at all hopeful.
- On fitting the confirmatory factor analysis item-wise, it was seen that all the factors except R8 (menstruation problems) had factor loading above 0.60 and were retained for the model for measuring physical well-being.
- The psychological well-being was measured through 17 items, and those with factor loading above 0.60 were selected for model fit. In all we have seven items that are extracted by the model, and they are R12 (deterioration in life quality), R13 (feeling of unhappiness), Psy15 (no satisfaction from life), R18 (appearance change), R21 (chemotherapy problems),

and R25 (anxiety). The ten items with factor loading less than 0.60 were deleted from the model. However, the fitness index in the model was achieved by examining the modification index (MI). The items with high correlation (MI >15) in the measurement errors were eliminated or they were set as a free parameter estimate from the correlated pair.

- The fearfulness (F3) construct was measured by five items, and the factor analysis was done for the same. All the items except Fr31 (feeling normal) had factor loading more than 0.60, and hence only Fr31 was deleted. **This factor has come to be the strongest factor contributing to quality of life.**

- The social well-being (F4) construct was measured by eight items, and the factor analysis was done for the same. We have only four items, viz; R36 (problem with job), R37 (problem with household activities), R38 (isolation), and R39 (financial burden) with strong negative feelings. To achieve fitness of the model the MI was examined, and the items with high correlation (MI >15) in the measurement errors were eliminated or they were set as a free parameter estimate from the correlated pair.

- The spiritual well-being (F5) construct is measured by seven items, but only three items, viz; Spr40 (religious activities), Spr41 (meditation), and Spr42 (spiritual change) were selected by the model after achieving the fitness index.

- After the confirmatory factor analysis (CFA) was conducted for all five constructs, the structural equation modelling (SEM) was done with the selected constructs.

- The correlation between the latent construct physical well-being and quality of life (QoL) is estimated to be 0.50. Thus, we can say that the physical parameters are responsible for 50% in deteriorating QoL.

- The psychological construct has only a 22.2% effect on QoL. This is because the third construct, fear, which was part of this construct in the measuring instrument is measured alone and contributed a lot to the QoL.

- The correlation between the latent construct fear and QoL is estimated to be 31%. This factor is contributing to a great extent, as most of the respondents reported that once cancer is detected, they live with the shadow of fear, and this is one of the major reasons for declining QoL.
- The social well-being construct contributes 67% to QoL. This is large because of the financial burden on patients and their relatives. Continuing to work becomes a problem.
- The spiritual well-being construct contributes 40% to QoL.

6.3 Scenario-2 Findings

- After undergoing treatment the respondents reported that the severity of various indicators like fatigue, appetite change, pain, sleep and weight change, constipation, nausea, menstrual change, etc., had reduce to some extent. Those suffering from grade IV cancer now only reported major physical problems like pain. Most respondents reported that treatment has been able to reduce their misery to a large extent (40%) and in some to a moderate level (35%). Thus we see that nearly 25% of the respondents have mild effects and the reason was that they were suffering from grade III or grade IV cancer.
- The psychological well-being parameter shows a great change after follow-up treatment, and respondents said that now they are able to cope with the disease or treatment. Anxiety and depression were reduced, and even the feelings of unhappiness and non-usefulness had reduced. Though there is no formal counselling cell for the cancer patients, doctors

at their individual level try to counsel patients on various problems they face.

- Thus we see the percentage drop in the patient category of 'not able to cope with the disease' reduced drastically (from 81.1% to 7.9%). The same scenario was apparent for 'difficulty in coping with treatment' (from 81.7% to 11.65%). The main reason was counselling by doctors and family members. The symptoms of severe anxiety and depression reduced from 78.8% and 78.5% to 13.53% and 16.54%, respectively. The feeling of unhappiness reduced drastically from 70.8% to 21.81%.
- Thus we see from Table 23 that fear is playing a very vital role in cancer patients. Nearly 90% of the patients were in fear of either recurrence of cancer or spreading of cancer; this percentage reduced to 9%. The fear of a second cancer reduced from 87.5% to 10.15%. Fear of future tests reduced from 85% to 9.02%.
- Nearly 72.4% of the patients reported that cancer has very adversely hampered their household activities, but after treatment and follow-up, this reduced to 16.92%.
- The effect on patients' jobs reduced from 67.9% to 34.22% after follow-up and treatment. The financial burden remained more or less the same, as cancer treatment is costly.
- The effect on sex life reduced from 66% to 25.94%. In both scenarios, family distress remained the same. The feeling of isolation reduced from 56.4% to 30.83%.
- Around 28.20% reported on the high uncertainty of their future, which was around 67% at the initial stage of cancer detection.
- Nearly 36.2% of patients said that prayer and meditation are highly important for them now, and this increased to 45.14%.
- Religious activities also increased mildly. Hopefulness in life increased from 29.2% to 53.76%.

- On fitting the CFA item-wise, it was seen that all the factors except R8 (menstruation problems) had factor loading above 0.60 and were retained for the model for measuring physical well-being. However, the fitness index was achieved by deleting R6 from the model.

- The psychological well-being (F2) construct was measured by 17 items, and the factor analysis was done for the same. Figure 14 shows the factor loading for each item for the psychological well-being latent exogenous variable. The item with factor loading above 0.60 had both positive feeling and negative feeling. To get better effective results, both are analysed. In all we have eight items that are extracted by the model. We have three items, viz; R12, R13, and R18 with a positive feeling, as seen in the Figure 14, whereas we have five items, viz; Psy14, Psy15, Psy16, Psy17, and Psy19, that have a negative feeling. The nine items with factor loading less than 0.60 will be deleted from the model. But to achieve model fitness, we have to introduce R18 with loading less than 0.6 but highest in the eliminated group.

- The fearfulness (F3) construct was measured by five items, and the factor analysis was done for the same. All the items except Fr31 had factor loading more than 0.60, and hence only Fr31 was deleted. The model fitness index was also achieved.

- The social well-being (F4) construct was measured by eight items, and the factor analysis was done for the same. We have only three items, viz; R37, R38, and R39 with a negative feeling. The remaining five items having factor loading less than 0.60 and were deleted from the model. To achieve the fitness index, we introduced Soc32 in the model.

- The spiritual well-being (F5) construct was measured by seven items, and the factor analysis was done for the same. We have four items, viz; Spr40, Spr41, Spr42, and Spr45 selected by the model, and the three items with factor loading less than 0.60 were deleted from the model. To achieve model fitness, we eliminated R43, Spr44, and Spr46 from the model.

■ After the selection of relevant exogenous variables through CFA, the next step was to proceed with SEM. The model is specified until unidimensionality for the model was achieved through fitness checking. The variables Psy15 and R25 were deleted from construct F2. R37 and R38 were deleted from construct F4. Spr44 was deleted from construct F5. After deleting these exogenous variables, the fitness indexes for the model were achieved.

■ It was estimated that QoL explains 93.0% of the variance, which means that the error variance of QoL is approximately 0.07% of the variance itself.

■ The correlation between the latent construct physical well-being and QoL was estimated to be 0.59. Thus, we can say that the physical parameters are responsible for 59% in deteriorating QoL.

■ The psychological construct had only a 22.2% effect on QoL in the initial stage but changed to 43% after follow-up and treatment. This is mainly because doctors along with relatives and friends have counselled patients positively with respect to their disease and they are now in better position to cope with it. Their anxiety and depression levels also reduced as a result of this.

■ The correlation between the latent construct fear and QoL is now estimated to be 25%, slightly less than the initial stage. This factor is contributing to a great extent, as most of the respondents reported that once cancer is detected, they live with the shadow of fear, and this is one of the major reasons in declining QoL. Now this suggest that if we open professional counselling cells in oncology departments just for these patients, we can overcome these fears to a great extent.

- The social well-being construct contributes 42% to QoL. This is mostly because of the financial burden on patients and their relatives. Continuing to work was a problem.
- The spiritual well-being construct contributes 40% to QoL and remained more or less the same in both scenarios.

6.4 Conclusion

The measurement of the QoL index assessment can assist with decision making and provide data in clinical trials and identify patients who need psychosocial interventions. As we see that mostly the low-income group are visiting these hospitals, they are more vulnerable to a low QoL, and cancer adds to their misery. Physical well-being primarily directly affects QoL from the start of the disease and after treatment also, but other factors are changing with treatment and follow-ups. Thus we see that non-professional counselling and treatment are the prominent factors that are reducing fear. There is a reduction in the fear factor and an increase in psychological well-being and social well-being factors. Before and after follow-up, no change was found in physical well-being because the physical symptoms remains more or less the same at the early stage of cancer and continues to deteriorate in the later stages of cancer. As the diagnosis and management of cancer can have a major impact on every aspect of a patient's QoL, this may benefit patients in terms of increasing their well-being.

6.5 Limitations and Recommendations

Limitations:

- Data, time, and money all were constrained in the present study.
- The same process, if studied for a longer period of time, could provide better results.

- The study was confined to one geographical location, but could be spread out to other areas for better results

Recommendations:

- There should be counselling centres for both the OPD and indoor patients suffering from cancer in the oncology department itself.
- There should be more research in this field in India, bringing out linkages with QoL and type of treatment, stage of disease, type of cancer, and long- and short-term effects of the disease.
- There should be time series and cross-sectional studies in the previously mentioned areas.
- Awareness programmes should be launched at a massive scale.

Bibliography

Akça, M., Ata, A., Nayir, E., Erdoğdu, S., and Arican, A. (2014). Impact of surgery type on quality of life in breast cancer patients. *The Journal of Breast Health*, 10 (4), 222.

Asadi Sadeghiazar, I., Vasudeva, P., and Abdollahi, A. (2006). Relationship between Quality of Life, hardiness, self-efficacy and self-esteem amongst employed and unemployed married women in Zabol. *Iranian Journal of Psychiatry*, 1 (3), 104–111.

Barrett, P. (2007). Structural equation modelling: Adjudging model fit. *Personality and Individual Differences*, 42 (5), 815–824.

Bentler, P. M. (1990). Comparative fit indexes in structural models. *Psychological Bulletin*, 107 (2), 238–246.

Blunch, N. J. (2012). *Introduction to Structural Equation Modeling using IBM SPS Statistics and AMOS.* 2nd edn. SAGE, 1–312.

Bollen, K. A. (1989). *Structural Equations with Latent Variables.* New York: John Wiley & Sons.

Brown, T. A. (2006). *Confirmatory Factor Analysis for Applied Research.* New York: The Guilford Press.

Browne, M. W., and Cudeck, R. (1993). Alternative ways of assessing model fit. In *Testing Structural Equation Models*, Bollen, K. A. and Long, J. S. Eds., pp. 136–162. Newbury Park, CA: SAGE.

Byrne, B. M. (2001). Structural equation modeling with AMOS, EQS, and LISREL: Comparative approaches to testing for the factorial validity of a measuring instrument. *International Journal of Testing*, 1 (1), 55–86.

Cha, K.-H. (2003). Subjective well-being among college students. *Social Indicators Research*, 62 (1), 455–477.

Chen, Y., Chen, M., Chou, F., Sun, F., Chen, P., and Tsai, K. (2007). The relationship between Quality of Life and posttraumatic stress disorder or major depression for firefighters in Kaohsiung, Taiwan. *Quality of Life Research*, 16 (8), 1289–1297.

Chow, H. P. H. (2005). Life satisfaction among university students in a Canadian prairie city: A multivariate analysis. *Social Indicators Research*, 70 (2), 139–150.

Dehkordi, A., Heydarnejad, M. S., and Fatehi, D. (2009). Quality of life in cancer patients undergoing chemotherapy. *Oman Medical Journal*, 24 (3), 204.

Disch, W. B., Harlow, L. L., Campbell, J. F., and Dougan, T. R. (2000). Student functioning, concerns, and socio-personal well-being. *Social Indicators Research*, 51 (1), 41–74.

D'Souza, P. J. J., Chakrabarty, J., Sulochana, B., and Gonsalves, J. (2013). Quality of life of head and neck cancer patients receiving cancer specific treatments. *Journal of Krishna Institute of Medical Sciences* (JKIMSU), 2 (1), 51–57.

Dubashi, B., Vidhubala, E., Cyriac, S., and Sagar, T. G. (2010). Quality of life among younger women with breast cancer: Study from a tertiary cancer institute in south India. *Indian Journal of Cancer*, 47 (2).

Echteld, M. A., van Zuylen, L., Bannink, M., Witkamp, E., and Van der Rijt, C. C. D. (2007). Changes in and correlates of individual Quality of Life in advanced cancer patients admitted to an academic unit for palliative care. *Palliative Medicine*, 21 (3), 199–205.

Elsaie, O. A., Elazazy, H. M., and Abdelhaie, S. A. (2012). The effect of chemotherapy on quality of life of colorectal cancer patients before and 21 days after the first chemotherapeutic sessions. *Life Science Journal*, 9 (4), 3505.

Ferlay, J., Soerjomataram, I., Dikshit, R., Eser, S., Mathers, C., Rebelo, M., Parkin, D. M., Forman, D., and Bray, F. (2015). Cancer incidence and mortality worldwide: Sources, methods and major patterns in GLOBOCAN 2012. *International Journal of Cancer*, 136 (5), E359–E386. doi: 10.1002/ijc.29210.

Ferrell, B. R., Dow, K. H., and Grant, M. (1995). Measurement of the Quality of Life in cancer survivors. *Quality of Life Research*, 4 (6), 523–531.

Ferrell, B. R., Dow, K. H., Leigh, S., Ly, J., and Gulasekaram, P. (1995). Quality of Life in long-term cancer survivors. *Oncology Nursing Forum*, 22 (6), 915–922.

GLOBOCAN, Global Cancer Observatory. (2014). World cancer factsheets 2014. IARC/WHO. Available at http://globocan.iarc.fr/Pages/fact_sheets_cancer.aspx (Assessed on 20 April 2019).

Government of India. (2012). 12th Five Year Plan (2012–2017). New Delhi Planning Commission.

Grace, J. B. (2006). *Structural Equation Modelling and Natural Systems*. Cambridge: Cambridge University Press.

Hagerty, M. R., Cummins, R. A., Ferriss, A. L., Land, K., Michalos, A. C., Peterson, M., Sharpe, A., Sirgy, M. J., and Vogel, J. (2001). Quality of Life indexes for national policy: Review and agenda for research. *Social Indicators Research*, 55 (1), 1–96.

Hair, J. F., Black, W. C., Babin, B. J., and Anderson, R. E. (2010). *Multivariate Data Analysis*. 7th edn. Upper Saddle River, NJ: Prentice Hall.

Hatcher, L. (2005). *A Step-By-Step Approach to Using SAS for Factor Analysis and Structural Equation Modeling*. Cary, NC: SAS Institute Inc.

Hemavathy, V., and Julius, A. (2016). A study to assess the quality of life among women with cervical cancer in selected hospitals at Chennai. *International Journal of Pharma and Bio Sciences*, 7 (4), 722–724.

Hoyle, R. H. (1995). *Structural Equation Modeling: Concepts, Issues, and Applications*. Thousand Oaks, CA: SAGE.

Hu, L. T., and Bentler, P. M. (1999). Cutoff criteria for fit indexes in covariance structure analysis: Conventional criteria versus new alternatives. *Structural Equation Modeling*, 6 (1), 1–55.

James, W. P. T., Ferro-Luzzi, A., and Waterlow, J. C. (1988). Definition of chronic energy deficiency in adults: Report of a working party of the international dietary energy consultative group. *European Journal of Clinical Nutrition* 42, 969–981.

Jöreskog, K. G. (1993). Testing structural equation models. In *Testing Structural Equation Models*, Bollen, K. A. and Lang, J. S. Eds., pp. 294–316. Newbury Park, CA: SAGE.

Jöreskog, K. G., and Sörbom, D. (1982). Recent developments in structural equation modeling. *Journal of Marketing Research*, 19 (4), 404–416.

Jöreskog, K. G., and Sörbom, D. (1986). *LISREL VI: Analysis of Linear Structural Relationships by Maximum Likelihood and Least Square Methods*. Mooresville, IN: Scientific Software, Inc.

Kannan, G., Rani, V., Ananthanarayanan, R. M., Palani, T., Nigam, N., Janardhan, V., and Reddy, U. M. (2011). Assessment of quality of life of cancer patients in a tertiary care hospital of South India. *Journal of Cancer Research and Therapeutics*, 7 (3), 275–279.

Kelloway, E. K. (1998). *Using LISREL for Structural Equation Modeling: A Researcher's Guide*. Thousand Oaks, CA: SAGE.

Kline, R. (2005). *Principles and Practices of Structural Equation Modelling*. 2nd edn. New York: Guilford Press.

Layard, R. (2007). Rethinking public economics: The implications of rivalry and habit. In *Economics & Happiness: Framing the Analysis*, Bruni, L. and Porta, P. L. Eds., pp. 147–170. New York: Oxford University Press.

Madhusudhan, C., Saluja, S. S., Pal, S., Ahuja, V., Saran, P., Dash, N. R., Sahni, P., and Chattopadhyay, T. K. (2009). Palliative stenting for relief of dysphagia in patients with inoperable esophageal cancer: Impact on Quality of Life. *Diseases of the Esophagus*, 22 (4), 331–336.

Mallath, M., Taylor, D. G., Badwe, R. A., Rath, G. K., Shanta, V., Pramesh, C. S., and Sullivan, R. (2014). The growing burden of cancer in India: epidemiology and social context. *Lancet Oncology*, 15 (6), e205–e212.

Mohamadkhani, K., Ghasemizad, A., and Kazemi, M. (2011). A study of factors influencing high school students' Quality of Life. *International Journal of Management and Business Research*, 1 (2), 53–58.

Mohd Zainudin, N. H., Mohd Radzi, J., AI, W., and SNI, I. (2012). Surface contamination in skin and room during hospitalization of thyroid cancer patient receiving radioiodine ablation. *IOSR Journal of Dental and Medical Sciences*, 2 (1), 27–33.

Patiño Pacheco, J. H., Agudelo, L. H. L., García Rúa, L. F., Agudelo, I. C. P., and Tatis, J. G. (2005). Quality of Life of patients with malignant obstruction of the esophagus, the bile ducts and the urinary tract after palliative radiological interventions. *Iatreia*, 18 (2), 141–159.

Saad, I. A. B., José Botega, N., and Contrera Toro, I. F. (2007). Predictors of Quality-of-Life improvement following pulmonary resection due to lung cancer. *Sao Paulo Medical Journal*, 125 (1), 46–49.

Santangelo, A., Testai, M., Barbagallo, P., Manuele, S., Di Stefano, A., Tomarchio, M., Trizzino, G., Musumeci, G., Panebianco, P., and Maugeri, D. (2006). The use of bisphosphonates in palliative treatment of bone metastases in a terminally ill, oncological elderly population. *Archives of Gerontology and Geriatrics*, 43 (2), 187–192.

Sewall, W. (1923). The theory of path coefficients. *Genetics*, 8, 238–255.

Srivastava, A., Tiwari, S., Chandra, G., and Shaswat (2019). Importance of counseling: Predicting Quality of Life of cancer patients in state of Uttar Pradesh. *Periyar Journal of Research in Business and Development Studies*, 4 (2), 29–38.

Srivastava, A., Tiwari, S., Chandra, G., and Shaswat. (2021). A vital analysis of factors affecting QoL in cancer patients in Uttar Pradesh through structural equation modelling approach. *International Journal of Behavioural and Healthcare Research*, 7 (4), 318–330.

Srivastava, S., Srivastava, A., and Tiwari, S. (2020). Factors affecting Quality of Life (QoL) in Breast Cancer Patients: A Case Study at King George's Medical University, Lucknow. *International Journal of Nursing Education*, 12 (4), 237–241.

Srivastava, S., Srivastava, A., and Tiwari, S. (2021). Low Quality of Life (QoL) in Indian breast cancer patients: A critical analysis of UP. *European Journal of Molecular & Clinical Medicine*, 7 (10), 1561–1575.

Srivastava, S., Srivastava, A., Tiwari, S., and Mishra, A. K. (2019). Life quality index assessment in breast cancer patients. *Indian Journal of Surgical Oncology*, 1–7.

Vidhubala, E., Kannan, R. R., Mani, C. S., Karthikesh, K., Muthuvel, R., Surendran, V., and Premkumari, R. (2005). Validation of Quality of Life questionnaire for patients with cancer–Indian scenario. *Indian Journal of Cancer*, 42 (3), 138.

Index

Note: Page numbers in *italics* indicate a figure and page numbers in **bold** indicate a table on the corresponding page.